Group CBT for Psychosis

Group CBT for Psychosis

A Guidebook for Clinicians

Tania Lecomte

WITH

Claude Leclerc and Til Wykes

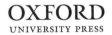

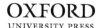

OXFORD
UNIVERSITY PRESS

Oxford University Press is a department of the University of Oxford. It furthers
the University's objective of excellence in research, scholarship, and education
by publishing worldwide. Oxford is a registered trade mark of Oxford University
Press in the UK and certain other countries.

Published in the United States of America by Oxford University Press
198 Madison Avenue, New York, NY 10016, United States of America.

Library of Congress Cataloging-in-Publication Data
Names: Lecomte, Tania, 1970– , author. | Leclerc, Claude, 1953– , author. |
Wykes, Til, author.
Title: Group CBT for psychosis : a guidebook for clinicians / Tania Lecomte,
with Claude Leclerc and Til Wykes.
Description: Oxford ; New York : Oxford University Press, [2016] | Includes
bibliographical references and index.
Identifiers: LCCN 2016005539 | ISBN 9780199391523 (alk. paper)
Subjects: | MESH: Cognitive Therapy—methods | Psychotic Disorders—therapy |
Psychotherapy, Group—methods
Classification: LCC RC489.C63 | NLM WM 425.5.C6 | DDC 616.89/1425—dc23
LC record available at http://lccn.loc.gov/2016005539

Contents

Introduction

The purpose of this book is to make group cognitive behavioral therapy (CBT) for psychosis more accessible to clinicians everywhere. Cognitive behavioral therapy for psychosis is now recognized as an evidence-based intervention that should be offered to whoever demands it. The limited number of psychologists who are trained in CBT for psychosis, along with the limited number of psychologists in general working with people with psychosis, have led us to develop the first published group workbook for CBT for psychosis that can be administered by mental health staff, not solely by psychologists. Our workbook has been empirically validated in rigorous studies and has obtained very strong empirical support, with participants also recognizing significant clinical improvements. Although the workbook is straightforward, clinicians typically need to have prior experience in group therapy, as well as a good knowledge of CBT principles and techniques, in order to run our CBT group for psychosis. For more than a decade now we have been teaching clinicians the skills necessary to run group CBT for psychosis; this book is an addition to that training and provides clinicians access to more information and guidance on the techniques that work.

The current book is based on years of experience in running groups with people with psychosis, particularly CBT for psychosis groups. The workbook and the various clinical examples should enable more clinicians working with individuals with psychosis to successfully conduct group CBT for psychosis. Although some clinicians will need more extensive training, this book should help all clinicians understand how group CBT for psychosis works, what are the essential therapeutic elements involved, and how to apply this group in their setting. It is meant as both a reference and a guidebook.

Group CBT for Psychosis

History of Group Therapies for People With Psychosis

Group interventions have been offered in institutionalized settings for many decades. This chapter reviews the changes in goals and purposes for group therapies over the years, describing psychoanalytical groups, encounter groups, milieu therapy, skills training, cognitive remediation groups, and peer support, to name a few.

Early Days: Psychoanalytical Group Therapy

Group interventions for people with psychotic disorders started many years ago, as early as 1921, when Edward W. Lazell began giving lectures to groups of patients in a psychiatric hospital in Washington, DC. Although these first groups mostly aimed at providing information, Lazell soon realized they also improved socialization of the participants. He later added discussions to his groups to further improve the participants' social skills. A few years later, as Sigmund Freud's ideas were becoming more popular worldwide, Lazell, along with psychoanalysts such as Wilfred Bion, Siegmund Heinz Foulkes, and Tom Main in England, applied the psychoanalytical principles to groups of inpatients and outpatients. The group in itself was viewed as a healing mechanism. In this model, psychosis was considered a personality structure that was ill-adapted as a result of inappropriate childhood interpersonal experiences (mostly interactions with parents were seen as the cause). The group would serve as a way to create positive relationships, repairing the harm caused by an inadequate family. The therapists believed that a healthy family-like setting, such as a therapeutic group, would allow participants to revisit their past in a safe way and address interpersonal problems through interactions with other participants and interpretations from the therapists (who were somewhat like the "parents" of the group).

Although these initial group therapies were developed with good intentions, and often resulted in increased socialization, critics (e.g., Gabrovsek, 2009) mention several limitations to their efficacy, particularly for individuals with psychotic disorders. For one, most psychoanalysts had been trained in individual analysis, primarily with individuals with neurosis, and simply tried to superimpose that model onto groups with psychosis. For instance, the analytical group was based on interpreting transference; it encouraged free association, with each member of the group being the "object" of the treatment, and every interaction in the group being subject to interpretation. Such groups when offered to people who had paranoid thoughts, who were socially anxious and withdrawn, or to people who presented with concrete thinking could quickly create even more confusion and anxiety, given the paucity of structure within the sessions. Lack of clear structure and goals in an inpatient group setting with people with psychosis quickly led to chaos, with participants accusing each other of being someone in their delusion (the Devil, for example). Another issue was related to the transference interpretations themselves: An individual with psychosis could experience them as intrusive and potentially dangerous, seeing the therapist as attempting to "steal his or her thoughts," for instance. Similarly, the focus on emotional expression often backfired, with participants not always being able to identify their emotions or easily becoming overwhelmed by others' emotional expression, therefore creating even more anxiety in attending the group (Gabrovsek, 2009).

Furthermore, given that there was little training available in group therapy at the time, many therapists "improvised," offering group sessions based on what they had read about or thought could be useful. Psychoanalytical group therapy for people with psychosis as described here is rarely seen anymore. Structured brief psychodynamic group approaches, involving interactive and dynamic therapists and with clearly defined goals for the group, can be found in some settings. Few studies, however, have been published to date that do or do not support these groups with individuals with psychosis.

Artistic Groups and Psychodrama

As psychoanalytical theory became the essential framework in most psychiatric hospitals, mental health clinicians explored various forms of treatments that could unleash the unconscious and help individuals with psychosis build better defense mechanisms through interpretation of their transcending unconscious thoughts. Art was considered by many as an efficient way to access the unconscious, particularly among patients with psychotic disorders who did not communicate much and were not good candidates for verbal therapy. Art therapy groups were created in which inpatients were asked to draw whatever came to mind and were then asked to describe the picture, ideally trying to think of what it reminded them of. Although this was often done in a group, the interventions were mostly individual, with the group used simply as the format for offering this therapy. Some art therapy groups allowed participants to expose their art, helping some of them to develop a sense of pride and of belonging to the group of "artists." Benefits to expressing oneself through art and improvements in self-esteem from exposing one's artistic creations have been reported; the usefulness of interpretation of such artworks for improving the person's well-being or alleviating symptoms has not been empirically demonstrated to date.

Another psychoanalytically inspired artistic group intervention is psychodrama. Developed by Jacob Moreno in 1925, it involved using theater, especially improvisation and multiple characters, to act out one's personal difficulties onstage. Various techniques were used, at times having multiple actors playing different facets of the same person, or having many actors playing the same person in the same situation, or having the person play different characters in his or her scenario. These variants aimed at helping the person understand the interpersonal issues at play and find ways to modify them. Psychodrama was always done in groups, often on a real stage with real prompts, but Moreno did not consider it group therapy because the focus was on one individual at a time. Sociodrama, a modified version of psychodrama, in contrast, is considered one of the early forms of group psychotherapy given that group issues and relationships that affected everyone in the group were played out (Bour, 1983). Moreno did not specifically target people in psychiatric institutions for his psychodrama, but several clinicians after him have done so. According to a fairly recent review (Ruddy & Dent-Brown, 2007), none of the studies using psychodrama or sociodrama with people with psychosis demonstrated evidence of benefits, not even in increased attendance compared with treatment as usual. Still, no studies have clearly demonstrated harm either.

Milieu Therapy

As new forms of treatments for people with mental illness emerged, groups often played an important part. For instance, the 1950s saw the development of the idea of a therapeutic community, where people with severe mental illness and mental health workers lived together as a small community, voting for rules and changes, and where everything in the environment was perceived as therapeutic (PsychiatricNursing, 2011). In such settings, groups were used for support and encouragement, for decision-making, and also for the influence of peer pressure on changing inappropriate behaviors—bringing (through feedback) the person to fit the group's social norm. Milieu therapy encouraged autonomy and aimed at improving adaptive coping skills through positive interactions. These groups offered the first opportunity for people with mental illness to have a voice in their treatment. Milieu therapy offered a context in which problematic behaviors could be addressed directly, and often successfully (Townsend et al., 2010). Unfortunately, such environments implied the quasi absence of hierarchy, a difficult concept to implement in a psychiatric setting. It was also difficult to adapt the environment to fit each person's needs, both at the inpatient level and in the community. In fact, milieu therapy is scarcely offered today, but the essence of its ideas can be found in the current recovery movement. Indeed, milieu therapy brought forth the idea of personal choice, of the person's own expertise regarding his or her mental health, of the beneficial role of having a job and of being an important member of one's community (PsychiatricNursing, 2011).

Encounter Groups

The encounter group grew exponentially more popular during the 1960s and 1970s, both in the general population and in clinical settings. In fact, most psychology or psychiatry students in those decades were required to attend such groups as part of their curriculum. The encounter group was a form of experiential group where participants' interactions were openly discussed in the here and now and where the goal was personal growth. Initially coming from social psychology and educational backgrounds, therapists were typically trained briefly, over a weekend, mostly in observing interactions and offering feedback. Very much influenced by Carl Rogers's humanistic movement, encounter groups aimed at inducing changes in self-actualization by addressing behaviors, attitudes, and values in the present moment. The encounter group was based on honesty but also on exploration, emotional expression, self-disclosure, and interpersonal confrontation. The effects of such groups were often linked to the leader's therapeutic style, with personnal attacks and overintrusive leaders having more dropouts or "casualties," that is, negative effects from the group (Yalom & Lieberman, 1971). Some leaders followed what Yalom and Leszcz (2005) describe as the "more is better" paradigm whereby participants were asked to interact in extreme ways. For instance, emotional expression could be pushed to the point of screaming and punching pillows; feedback could become incessant verbal attacks from group members until the person broke down crying; revealing personal secrets could be asked but naked, to truly show oneself. Many versions of encounter groups appeared during those years, with a subsample of participants experiencing "decompensation" or psychotic episodes as a result. Although leaders of encounter groups in the community rejected references to illness or symptoms, contrasting their "mind-opening" techniques to "head shrinking" by psychiatrists or trained clinicians, the essence of such experiential groups did translate into clinical settings, namely, in psychiatric institutions and outpatient services offered to people with psychosis. Well-trained Rogerian encounter group leaders in psychiatric settings mostly offered empathy and understanding and tried to help people grow by focusing on positive here-and-now interactions, limiting harsh confrontations, and they typically did not report important casualties. However, no studies have reported any benefits from encounter groups with people with psychosis. In fact, although they might be considered as predecessors of Irvin Yalom's interpersonal group approach or Nick Kanas's integrated approach, encounter groups are rare and are no longer offered to people with psychosis.

Yalom's Inpatient Interpersonal Group Approach

Irvin Yalom's book *The Theory and Practice of Group Psychotherapy*, initially published in 1970 and now in its fifth edition, is still in many ways considered the bible of group therapy. The book covers in detail years of research on the essential elements of group therapy, many of them being described in the current book in cognitive or behavioral terms in Chapter 4. Yalom's own theoretical model or theoretical influences are never thoroughly or clearly described, though psychodynamic, existential, and social learning theories are evident in his work. His interpersonal approach aims at providing a corrective experience to heal early traumatic experiences, linking past experiences with the here and now and using the positive group interactions as social learning. As in Rogerian encounter groups, empathy, expression of emotions happening in the present, and therapist transparency (e.g., the therapist disclosing his or her own feelings during interactions) are encouraged. Yalom's approach also focuses on early childhood experiences, with the group being perceived as a corrective family and transference at times being interpreted, as in the psychoanalytic approach. Yalom's interest in research lay mostly with process variables, focusing on facilitators of change. Through his empirical work and clinical experience, he describes therapeutic factors that are essential in order for a group therapy to induce change. These are instillation of hope, universality, imparting information, altruism (a desire to help others), interpersonal learning, group cohesiveness, development of socializing techniques, corrective family re-enactment, and imitative behavior. Many of these elements are present in evidence-based group interventions and have been demonstrated in empirical studies, such as group cohesion (Norcross & Wampold, 2011) and universality (or normalization), whereas others have yet to be demonstrated as essential (e.g., the corrective family re-enactment).

Yalom has worked for many years with people with psychiatric disorders in inpatient settings and has described important factors to consider when working with this population, ranging from organizational barriers to the importance of providing structure and formulating clear goals for the therapy (Yalom, 1983). However, unlike behavioral or cognitive behavioral group therapists, he does not believe that important changes can occur with this clientele over a short period of time and proposes instead that the therapy should simply aim at getting people to talk, become less isolated, and attempt to be helpful to others.

Kanas's Integrated Model

Like Yalom, Nick Kanas (1996) has devoted much time to studying process issues in group psychotherapy but focusing almost exclusively on people with psychosis. His approach is influenced by Yalom's work, incorporating psychodynamic, interpersonal, and existential components but also adding psychoeducation and advice giving into the model.

The group's aim, in Kanas's approach, is to help people develop coping strategies for their symptoms and find solutions to interpersonal difficulties they might share. Based on his studies, he has proposed certain guidelines when working with people with psychosis in group psychotherapy, particularly in inpatient settings: Groups should be homogeneous in terms of diagnosis (this point will be addressed in more detail in Chapter 6, with a slightly different twist), groups that focus on interpersonal aspects work better than groups that aim at improving insight in the psychoanalytical sense, emotional expression is encouraged but excludes the expression of anger, and reality testing is encouraged. Unlike other therapists of the time, Kanas encouraged the expression and description of delusional thoughts, as well as exploring ways to determine if the patient's experience was based in reality or not. Some of the principles and techniques used by Kanas are also found in cognitive behavioral therapy (CBT) for psychosis, namely, openly discussing symptoms and checking the facts (see Chapter 8). Kanas also used the group as a platform to improve social interactions and practice social skills—something behaviorists greatly developed—even encouraging participants to interact outside the group.

Skills Training

As the golden age of psychiatric institutions passed, individuals needed to be prepared to return to the community, often after having spent many years incarcerated in psychiatric asylums. Clinicians quickly realized that psychoeducation training, often resembling classes, giving verbal instructions and information regarding the effects of medication and the importance of adherence, for instance, did not suffice. In fact, psychoeducation training rarely enabled behavioral changes and often addressed only topics pertaining to the illness or to medication, whereas many other behaviors needed to be mastered in order to lead fulfilling community lives. Behavioral group interventions became essential. Based on Albert Bandura's theory of self-efficacy, interventions were tailored to optimize learning through the demonstration of appropriate social behaviors, repetition, and social encouragement. Skills training, namely, independent living skills and social skills, was offered in groups using Bandura's self-efficacy model. Individuals learned most of the skills in groups, including how to cook simple meals, how to start a friendly conversation with a neighbor, and how to be happy and satisfied at work. Two pioneers in social skills training were Robert Liberman and Charles Wallace, from the University of California, Los Angeles. In the 1980s and early 1990s they developed and studied (often in randomized controlled trials) a large array of modules and videos for skills training (see www.psychiatricrehab.com). Some skills were more medically oriented, such as learning to independently manage one's medication or to recognize and cope with one's symptoms, whereas others were more social (e.g., skills for developing friendship and intimacy). A number of books have been written on social skills training (e.g., Bellack, Mueser, Gingerich, & Agresta, 2004; Liberman, 1992), but they essentially include the same recipe: (a) Introduce the skill to be learned (why is it important to learn this skill?); (b) demonstrate how to apply the skill (model it or show a video); (c) practice the skill (role plays with feedback); (d) plan the needed resources to use the skill; (e) do it! (in vivo); (f) if things do not work as planned, use problem-solving; and (g) try again (independently).

It is important to mention that each large skill is broken down into smaller skills that are easier to learn. For instance, learning how to take medication autonomously can be divided into several skills: (a) how to verify your prescription and dosage; (b) how to count your pills and remember to take them daily; (c) how to record side effects and discuss them with your doctor at your next appointment.

In a group setting, social skills training would involve everyone reading and learning together about a new skill. For example, for the skill "how to record side effects and discuss them with your doctor," after learning about the skill, the participants would see an example (such as a video recording) of someone having tracked on a sheet daily side effects and showing it to his or her doctor while saying that he or she is really bothered by one specific side effect. This would be followed by a group discussion regarding what the group members saw and understood in the video. Then participants would be asked to recognize their own side effects, using the same tracking sheet as was seen in the video. This could also be done as a take-home assignment. The following group session would involve participants role-playing either the client or the doctor, with the client trying to explain to the doctor his or her preoccupation with a specific side effect. Everyone else in the group would be instructed to notice verbal and nonverbal signs such as tone, eye contact, posture, and the coherence of the message conveyed. Following a role play, positive and constructive feedback is always offered before comments on aspects that need improvement. Everyone would get a turn at trying the new skill in a role play, with participants at times doing the role play many times in a row to get it right. The following sessions would explain the seven steps in problem-solving, which are as follows:

- Is there a problem?
- What is the problem?
- What are potential solutions?
- What are pros and cons for each solution?
- Which solution seems the best at this point?
- Verify resources.
- Do it!

The participants would be instructed to come up with examples of what might go wrong when trying to apply, for instance, the skill "how to record side effects and discuss them with your doctor." Each potential problem would be a target for the seven-step problem-solving technique. Discussions pertaining to the resources needed to apply the skill and how to practice the skill outside of the group before meeting the doctor would also take place. Finally, actual applications of the skill in real life would take place, with participants coming back to the group for feedback. Such behavioral groups are time-limited, with an average of 24 sessions for skills such as the medication management skills illustrated here. These groups usually end with a graduation party, where a diploma is given to each graduating participant and a friendly meal is served. Studies have demonstrated that social skills training in groups does improve the actual learning of the skill and, when offered in conjunction with community support, can lead to sustained learning (Kopelowicz, Liberman, & Zarate, 2006). Social skills training was essential during the deinstitutionalization era but is still used today, especially with individuals who have poor social skills and cognitive deficits. In fact, many group cognitive remediation programs for people with cognitive deficits include social skills training.

Cognitive Skills Groups

Along with social skills training, the 1980s were marked by the arrival of more comprehensive assessments of neurocognitive impairments in individuals with schizophrenia. Specific deficits in subtypes of memory or attention were documented, along with deficits in other aspects of executive functioning. A group of clinicians and researchers from Germany developed a stepwise group program, known as *integrated psychological therapy* (IPT), keeping in mind these deficits in order to teach participants how to improve their cognitive skills (Roder, Mueller, Mueser, & Brenner, 2006). Given the perceived importance of these skills for social functioning, the program also included social skills training at the end, as the ultimate skills to master. Initially available in inpatient settings, IPT was offered in groups from two to five times a week for up to 12 months. The program covered basic cognitive skills (e.g., remembering elements on a card), more complex language skills (synonyms and antonyms, or synthesizing information), and more complex social problem-solving. Eventually, it also included more social cognitive elements of emotional recognition and regulation (Roder et al., 2006). The groups focused on learning new skills, not on group processes, and therapists were instructed to offer the information in the most neutral way possible (until they reached the social skills training part). A meta-analysis describes this group intervention as being effective in improving cognitive skills, especially when offered together with skills training, but does not offer evidence that it actually improves functioning (Roder et al., 2006). Although IPT is still offered in various community or outpatient settings today, the authors themselves do not recommend it for people with early psychosis given the length of the treatment.

Since this first cognitive skills group, other groups aiming at improving cognitive skills along with social skills have been developed and studied, with most being offered as an adjunct to individual cognitive remediation, such as computer training (McGurk, Mueser, & Pascaris, 2005) or even attempting to modify cognitive biases that underlie specific psychotic symptoms, using metacognitive training (MCT; Moritz et al., 2011). *Metacognition* here refers to abilities linked to social cognitive skills such as theory of mind, as well as judgment skills such as not jumping to conclusions, or appropriately determining timelines or attributing causal links in cartoon storyboards, for instance. Such groups offer validated training that in several pilot studies has demonstrated preliminary evidence for its potential for improving metacognitive skills (Moritz et al., 2011). Both MCT and IPT are considered more "training" than "therapy" given that personal problems and goals are not brought up, and group processes are not acknowledged.

Peer-Support Groups

Peer support comes in many formats and has changed greatly over the years (Davidson, Chinman, Sells, & Rowe, 2006). Already in the 1970s, individuals with mental illness living in the community wished to benefit from sharing and meeting with people with similar difficulties. Various groups that aimed at offering support in a nonstigmatizing environment, free of medical staff, were developed and led by people with mental illness, for people with mental illness. Clubhouses, such as Fountain House in New York City, offered groups that met weekly over coffee and snacks. The discussions were often informal, but at times they could address a specific theme, depending on what participants wanted. Today these support groups are usually open, with newcomers always welcome, and time-unlimited. The therapeutic elements in these groups are mostly social support and belonging, given the absence of clear goals or tools. Attendees mention developing friendships, feeling similar to others in the group, and being able to share their experiences without being judged. Peer-support groups are considered useful mostly for social reasons, given that many who attend are otherwise socially isolated. However, the therapeutic value of these groups is limited by the absence of therapists, of goals, and of tools to help with any of the issues that are brought up. For instance, groups for individuals who hear voices exist in a few countries and enable people to share their experience, providing self-help but without offering evidence-based strategies to alleviate the voices or help individuals feel more in control of the voices (although such strategies have been demonstrated in CBT for psychosis, for instance; Wykes, Parr, & Landau, 1999). Similarly, groups based on the Alcoholics Anonymous framework, such as Schizophrenia Anonymous or Dual Diagnosis Anonymous, offer steps to follow and gatherings that help instill hope and help participants feel more connected with others and less lonely, but they do not offer a group therapy context per se and do not really help people deal with their personal issues. As such, peer-support groups that operate in the traditional way (reciprocal relationships, no therapist) are not considered group therapy and have not yielded any specific benefits in studies other than the ones mentioned here. They do, however, offer a setting where participants can meet people with similar issues and potentially make friends.

There is today another form of peer-run therapeutic groups that stems from the recovery movement whereby peers with training and sufficient expertise can become mental health therapists and offer various services, from case management to psychotherapy, including group psychotherapy (Davidson et al., 2006). The peer worker is not simply someone who is further along in his or her recovery and can testify that things can get better, but is someone who has experienced psychosis firsthand and also obtained the needed qualifications to become a therapist. Such peer workers not only can offer effective interventions such as group CBT for psychosis but also can offer hope and serve somewhat as role models, given their experience with the mental health system. Studies have compared outcomes of clients followed in case management by a peer worker versus another mental health worker and to date have not found any significant differences, with some studies finding slightly higher community tenure for the former (Davidson et al., 2006). No study to date, however, has examined the impact of peer mental health therapists offering group therapy, such as CBT for psychosis. Should the therapists possess the necessary skills and attitudes, and master the model and principles, one can only expect that they could become efficient therapists for group CBT for psychosis.

Dual-Diagnosis Groups

One of the biggest problems that people with severe mental illness, including people with psychosis, face in the community is substance misuse. Substance abuse and dependence is reported to affect close to 50% of all individuals with a severe mental illness (Mueser, Drake, & Wallach, 1998). To help people quit or control their substance misuse, groups have been designed specifically for people with a dual diagnosis of both a severe mental illness and a substance misuse problem. These groups are mostly based on the substance abuse literature, using the stages of motivation and change framework (Prochaska, DiClemente, & Norcross, 1992), but they also include skills training and CBT techniques, although not CBT for psychosis specifically. Mueser and colleagues, in their book *Integrated Treatments for Dual Disorder* (2003), provide good examples of how people might initially take part in a group equivalent of motivational interviewing (called *persuasion groups*), where people are not confronted on their substance use but instead are brought to explore in an empathic and nonjudgmental way how their substance use is helping them (or not) reach their life goals. Once group members mention wishing to stop their substance misuse, they can move on to a more "active treatment" group where new skills are taught, coping strategies are shared, and alternative behaviors are practiced between group sessions. The dual-disorder groups aim at decreasing or stopping substance misuse and focus on psychotic symptoms only indirectly (i.e., as a potential consequence of substance misuse). It is very difficult for people with dual disorders to completely stop using drugs for many reasons, such as an increased sensitivity to the effects of the substance, and, for many, the social context of substance misuse. Some studies have shown the efficacy of dual-disorder groups, compared with more traditional treatments, on substance reduction, although more studies are warranted (Mueser, Deavers, Penn, & Cassisi, 2013).

Conclusion

Reviewing the history of group psychotherapy for people with severe mental disorders helps us recognize the central role that group psychotherapy and other group interventions have had over the years in working with this clientele. Therapists and clinicians quickly realized the value of bringing people together, not only for improved social support but also so they could gain from sharing experiences and coping strategies. Furthermore, in times of budget and time constraints, group psychotherapy becomes even more appealing because many individuals can be treated at once. History has taught us that participants in a group are in many ways co-therapists, sharing the group's functioning and success with the therapists. Group psychotherapy for people with mental illness has also gone through many phases, from unstructured formats that attempt to reach unconscious processes, to at times overly structured behavioral interventions, as well as multiple variants in between. Group CBT for psychosis has integrated the acquired knowledge from the various group interventions presented here to keep only the central and most active elements that can lead both to symptom reduction and to increased self-esteem and well-being.

Basic Cognitive Behavioral Model Used in Group CBT for Psychosis

This chapter reviews the essential CBT model, as well as the specifics linked to psychosis in terms of different core beliefs, either specific to psychosis or shared by other disorders such as depression. Cognitive and behavioral theories explaining positive symptoms[1] such as paranoia and grandiosity and negative symptoms are also presented. Other models used in group CBT for psychosis, such as the vulnerability-stress-competence model and the recovery model, are explained.

Basic Cognitive Behavioral Model Used in Most CBT Interventions

A. T. Beck developed his model for CBT in the 1950s and later refined it both clinically and empirically. Beck recognized a need for CBT after realizing that symptomatic change did not come quickly following simple realizations of past troubles but could be accelerated with changes in thinking patterns and behaviors. Cognitive behavioral therapy brought down to its simplest model is often described as the A-B-C model, although this model was initially presented by Albert Ellis (Wallen et al., 1992). The A-B-C model essentially illustrates that any thought or belief (B) is preceded by a situation or an antecedent (A), and that the belief will influence how one will feel and act as a consequence (C) (Figure 2.1).

1. In psychosis and in psychotic disorders such as schizophrenia, positive symptoms refer to symptoms that did not exist before the illness onset, such as delusions and hallucinations, whereas negative symptoms refer to behaviors or expressions that have been lost, such as lack of motivation, blunted emotions, lack of pleasure, to name a few.

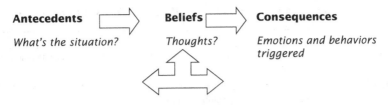

Antecedents   **Beliefs**   **Consequences**

What's the situation?   *Thoughts?*   *Emotions and behaviors triggered*

FIGURE 2.1 A-B-C of CBT.

What makes this an interesting model for change is that modifying any of the elements can produce a change in another. For instance, changing the belief will change the emotion and behaviors linked to the belief. A change in behavior also can change the situation, leading to new thoughts, new emotions, and new behaviors. For example, the situation A (no one talks to me at work), can bring you to believe B (everyone hates me), which in turn results C (makes you feel sad and brings you to withdraw). A change in B (new thought: maybe people are just really busy) or a change in C (new behavior: I say hi and share cupcakes I made with my colleagues) could lead to a change in the situation, with more people greeting you every day.

Another interesting aspect of the A-B-C model is that it also takes into consideration the "why": Why am I thinking this way? Where does this come from? Unlike psychoanalytical models for which that is the most important question, in CBT this question refers to past experiences that have helped create core beliefs the person holds about him- or herself and the world. The core belief overshadows many daily beliefs people hold. Beck, Rush, Shaw, and Emery (1979) defined three types of core beliefs: beliefs about the self, about others, and about the future. Some core beliefs are entrenched, extremely stable over time, and more difficult to change; these are called *schemas* by Jeffrey Young and colleagues (2003). When a core belief is negative, it can lead to specific cognitive biases and can alter the person's daily thinking, resulting in the person noticing only evidence that will confirm this belief and disregarding anything that might contradict it. Cognitive biases are somewhat like colored glasses, allowing the person to see things only in that color. Some people might have several cognitive biases, though these biases tend to all serve the same function, namely, to help prove that whatever thought the person holds that is creating distress is based on real facts and cannot be disputed.

Typically, people with depression will present with at least one of the following core beliefs: I am not capable of being loved (not lovable), or I am not able to face challenges (incompetent). These two core beliefs are linked to specific cognitive biases in depression as well (Table 2.1).

Certain cognitive biases can be found in more than one disorder. For instance, the cognitive biases described here have been linked to depression, but some are also found in individuals with psychosis, and not only because many concurrently experience depression (Wigman et al., 2012) or because the stigma associated with having a severe mental illness negatively modifies how one sees him- or herself and the world. In fact, some of

TABLE 2.1 Common cognitive biases found in people with depression

Cognitive Bias	Meaning
Overgeneralization	The smallest mistake the person makes is proof that he or she is incapable of anything.
Catastrophizing	Any small event (e.g., someone is late) is interpreted as something terrible (e.g., is not coming = must hate me).
Personalizing	This bias is linked to the concept of attribution and implies blaming oneself for everything, even accidents or events out of their control.
Arbitrary inference	This bias implies the person proves a point or comes to a conclusion based on insufficient information; it is also known as the jumping-to-conclusions bias.
Selective abstraction	It has been demonstrated in studies that people with depression can intentionally focus only on certain elements, namely, things that make them sad, and will ignore the rest. As such, they can minimize the information that contradicts their beliefs and magnify the importance of information that supports their beliefs.

these cognitive biases have been studied as specifically linked to paranoia or psychosis, for instance, arbitrary reference and selective abstraction.

This list of cognitive biases is not exhaustive, and others can be found in individuals with depression and those with other problems. Individuals with anxiety tend to have some similar biases as those with depression (in terms of pessimistic thinking), as well as a strong attentional bias toward threatening elements in the environment. Individuals with personality disorders, especially cluster B disorders, tend to have some of these as well (Table 2.2).

Specific Cognitive Behavioral Therapy Models for Psychosis

For some time now, schizophrenia has been understood as the interaction of genetic or biological predispositions and environmental stressors (Zubin & Spring, 1977). Although this stress-diathesis model has been used in many explanatory models for psychosis, and is used in a modified version in group CBT for psychosis, it did not open the door to offering CBT for psychosis.

TABLE 2.2 Common cognitive biases found in people with personality disorder

Cognitive Bias	Meaning
All-or nothing-thinking	Person sees things as black or white and people as good or bad, with no nuances or shades of gray.
Mind reading	Person is convinced that others hold opinions about him- or herself, based not on facts but on "intuition" or because they "know" how the other thinks.
Emotional reasoning	Similar to mind reading, this cognitive bias refers to the way a person is convinced of something because he or she "feels" it must be true or has a "gut feeling" or some other form of emotional intuition without any real tangible facts.
Labeling	Similar to personalization, this cognitive bias reflects the person's confusion between an action and a trait ("I made a stupid mistake, therefore I am a stupid person").

Cognitive behavioral therapy for psychosis in fact became a possible option following interesting results in cognitive psychology pertaining to the actual nature of psychotic symptoms such as hallucinations and delusions (Kingdon, Turkington, & John, 1994). Whereas symptoms such as delusions had been considered "empty speech acts, whose informational content refers to neither world nor self" (Berrios, 1991, p. 12) and, by definition, thoughts that were crystallized and impossible to change, studies in cognitive biases have led clinicians and researchers to believe otherwise. In fact, conviction or "absolute certainty" regarding a specific delusional belief can often fluctuate over time, leaving room for questioning or using strategies and techniques that might induce further doubts (Brett-Jones, Garety, & Hemsley, 1987). As such, a number of reasoning biases have been demonstrated in individuals presenting with abnormal beliefs. A well-documented judgment bias often found in people with delusions is the jumping-to-conclusions (JTC) bias (Garety, Hemsley, & Wessely, 1991), which resembles the arbitrary inference bias in that insufficient information is gathered prior to making a decision. The JTC bias is often documented by the bead task (or an equivalent: the fishing task) whereby a person is informed that two jars have inverse proportions of beads of black or white color (e.g., jar A has 60% white and 40% black; jar B has the opposite) and that the evaluator will be removing beads from a single jar, one at a time. The person needs to decide from which jar the beads are being removed, and tells the evaluator when he or she is sure regarding which of the two jars the beads are being removed from. People with active delusions will typically make a decision too quickly, after only a few beads but people without delusions typically wait until they have seen many more beads, before making a decision. Similarly, people who have become less delusional (for instance, they are not as convinced in their beliefs because they have received group CBT for psychosis) will show an improvement in this bias as well, gathering more evidence before making a decision (Woodward, Munz, Leclerc, & Lecomte, 2009).

Another bias concerns attributions. The concept of attribution was alluded to in regard to personalization in depression but can in fact include a few other cognitive biases as well. The bias refers to the explanations a person holds regarding experiences in his or her life, in terms of who might be responsible (self/internal or others/external), but also whether the experience is perceived as specific or global, and stable or temporary. For instance, a man notices a scratch on his car and thinks, "It must be my fault, I'm always such a terrible driver, a terrible person, I should never be allowed to drive." In this case, the accidental scratch is seen as internal (his fault), stable (always), and global (terrible driver = terrible person). We also notice that he personalized the accident, using labeling and overgeneralization. People with paranoia might hold somewhat opposite beliefs: Everything is always someone else's fault (Kinderman & Bentall, 2000). Table 2.3 represents different attributions for another situation, in this case a bad grade on an exam.

As can be seen from the table, external attributions can range from being slightly defensive or narcissistic to straight-out paranoid and delusional. People with psychosis and paranoia will tend to err on the side of overly attributing things they experience as being external. There are many potential reasons for this attributional bias. Some authors

TABLE 2.3 Examples of thoughts linked to specific attributional biases

	Internal	External
Unstable, specific	You were tired that morning.	This teacher is mad at you for asking tricky questions at the last class.
Unstable, global	You have been having a rough time since your girlfriend left you last week.	You have been so harassed by government people following you that you couldn't concentrate.
Stable, specific	You are not very good in multiple-choice exams.	Teachers always envy your intelligence and try to make you suffer for it.
Stable, global	You are really stupid.	There is a global conspiracy against you—this is further proof.

argue it might serve the purpose of protecting a fragile sense of self (Udachina, Varese, Oorschot, Myin-Germeys, & Bentall, 2013): If the person can do no wrong and in fact has great powers, and all the bad he or she experiences is because of others, he or she must have some internal value. It might be argued that the learning context also plays a role, whereby families who do not trust others and speak negatively of the government, for instance, might indirectly encourage an external attributional style that becomes even more apparent in psychosis. Nonetheless, attributional biases that are external and global, linked with other judgment biases such as jumping to conclusions too quickly, are found in people who are convinced that they are being threatened.

Attributional biases also apply to hallucinations. For instance, auditory hallucinations of individuals with psychosis are a form of external misattribution of their inner speech (Bentall & Slade, 1985; Hoffman, 1986). Most people are aware of their "inner speech," that is, the internal dialogues that they have throughout the day. This inner speech, and similarly auditory hallucinations, can even be detected by the activation of speech muscles (Stephane, Barton, & Boutros, 2001). These observations suggest that people who experience hallucinations have difficulties distinguishing between self-generated experiences and experiences stemming from the outside world (also called *source monitoring deficit*; Anselmetti et al., 2007). Other than the attributional bias of their voices being external, people with psychosis who hear voices often hold certain beliefs about their voices, such as beliefs that the voices have power over them (omnipotence) or that the voices know everything (omniscience) and can therefore control them (Birchwood, Meaden, Trower, Gilbert, & Plaistow, 2000).

Individuals with psychosis also hold core beliefs that are reflected in their cognitive biases. Some of these beliefs can resemble those found in people with depression, namely, the belief of being worthless, although it can be expressed in a different way. People with depression will say they are bad and worthless, whereas someone with psychosis might believe he has superpowers, a belief that masks an underlying core belief that he is worthless. Grandiosity can often indicate that the person holds a core belief about the self as unlovable or worthless. However, grandiosity is not always apparent, and some individuals might present paranoid fears of being kidnapped or having their organs removed that might also serve as a self-esteem protector for the core belief of being worthless (i.e., if people want you, or wish to take your organs, you must hold some value in their eyes).

Another core belief is that the world is a dangerous place. Given the high rate of childhood trauma in people with psychosis, it is unsurprising that many fear the world, and people in general, and constantly feel threatened. In fact, a recent plethora of studies have suggested that close to 35% of people with psychosis have experienced trauma (Bonoldi et al., 2013) and that childhood trauma increases the odds of developing psychosis by 2.8 times (Varese et al., 2012). Sexual trauma specifically has been linked with increased odds for auditory hallucinations (Bentall, Wickham, Shevlin, & Varese, 2012). A recently identified and perhaps more insidious form of trauma, bullying, has also been documented as greatly increasing one's odds of developing schizophrenia (Arseneault et al., 2011). The same group of researchers did, however, find that parental support could counteract the effects of bullying. Unfortunately, individuals who have experienced trauma as children often re-experience trauma as adults, resulting in higher rates of post-traumatic stress disorder (PTSD). This re-exposure to trauma can be partly explained by the family context (unsafe environments often stay unsafe,) as well as by the person's coping strategies. For instance, many individuals who have experienced trauma will eventually abuse substances such as street drugs or alcohol, often as a coping mechanism but also putting them at risk of being in situations where further traumatization is possible. In fact, a modified version of Mueser's supersensitivity model (Mueser, Rosenberg, Goodman, & Trumbetta, 2002) describes how past traumas and substance abuse make people more vulnerable to developing PTSD and psychosis (Figure 2.2).

Another important aspect of this model is that people with psychotic disorders, such as schizophrenia, in addition to psychotic symptoms also display depressive symptoms

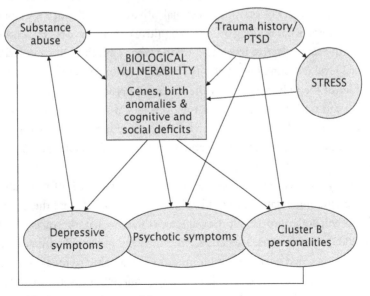

FIGURE 2.2 Modified supersensitivity model.

(Wigman et al., 2012), as mentioned previously, as well as substance abuse, symptoms of anxiety, or even symptoms of personality disorders. More than 50% of individuals with severe mental illnesses will present with substance abuse (Mueser et al., 1990). Studies have documented that close to 30% of individuals with schizophrenia also present with social anxiety (Lysaker & Salyers, 2007), suggesting that they not only believe the world is a dangerous place but also fear that others will judge them negatively. This belief could be linked to poor self-esteem, an attentional bias to threatening stimuli, difficulties in recognizing others' intentions and emotions (metacognitive deficits, described later), or experiences of stigmatization. Experiences of stigmatization are very common and contribute to already held beliefs regarding the person's worthlessness and his or her fears of rejection. Personality aspects are also mentioned in this model. For example, close to 30% of people with psychosis will present with a cluster B personality disorder, namely, narcissistic, borderline, antisocial, or histrionic (Wickett et al., 2006). Mostly borderline and antisocial personalities have been documented to date, which is not surprising given their common etiology of childhood trauma. In terms of cognitive biases, people with such personality traits tend to see the world as black or white. They also have multiple metacognitive deficits, namely, in recognizing others' mental states and in emotional regulation.

Studies are now suggesting that metacognitive and social cognitive deficits might help explain or further emphasize some of the biases mentioned earlier in this chapter. For instance, individuals with schizophrenia tend to have difficulties correctly identifying emotions in others, as well as recognizing thinking processes they or others might experience (Salvatore, Dimaggio, Popolo, & Lysaker, 2008). They also have difficulties recognizing their own emotional processes and self-regulating when confronted with stress (El-Khoury & Lecomte, 2012). These social and metacognitive deficits can lead people to mistrust others or fear interpersonal situations, given they are not capable of correctly identifying what is going on. Metacognitive deficits have been identified at various levels: at the self-reflective level (identifying what I am thinking and feeling), at the interpersonal level (recognizing what others can be feeling and thinking, and that I am not the center of the universe), and at the action or mastery level (given I know myself and others, I can find strategies to help me overcome difficulties I encounter). As with the JTC bias, most of these metacognitive biases are reduced as a person becomes less entrenched in his or her beliefs and is able to interact and reciprocate in interpersonal relationships (Lysaker et al., 2013).

As for negative symptoms, some authors suggest that lack of motivation, lack of pleasure, and emotional flatness might be linked to core beliefs that there is no point in trying, things will not improve, failure awaits, and therefore withdrawal is preferred (Beck & Rector, 2005). In this sense, negative symptoms are perceived as defeatist cognitive biases. Others argue that negative symptoms are a way of taking a break from the sensory overload of positive symptoms, somehow shutting oneself out of the overly frightening and chaotic emotional world (Hemsley, 1996). In many ways, negative symptoms can resemble depressive symptoms in motor retardation and lack of pleasure and goals, and they tend to improve in the same way as depression, that is, with set goals and behavioral activation (this will be discussed in more detail later).

Additional Models Used in Group CBT for Psychosis

Although group CBT for psychosis essentially uses the same models as individual CBT for psychosis, the group context encourages the use of models developed for psychiatric rehabilitation, namely, the recovery model and the vulnerability-stress-competence model. The *recovery model* is particularly relevant given that it is the predominant model of clinical care in psychiatry for people with psychosis. *Recovery* is, however, a fairly broad term that involves both subjective internal aspects, such as maintaining hope and developing a new sense of direction in life, and objective external aspects, namely, obtaining and keeping employment and independent housing (Noiseux et al., 2009). The scientific community is somewhat divided regarding what constitutes recovery from a severe mental illness (Silverstein & Bellack, 2008). Scientists seek tangible criteria or measures of recovery and have thus decided that recovery can be defined in terms of functioning and should involve 2 years with low psychotic symptoms, 50% of the time spent at work or school, independent management of finances and medication, and socialization with peers at least once a week (Liberman & Kopelowicz, 2005). Recovery as seen from the consumer-survivor movement, in contrast, is defined as a personal journey through various stages (moratorium or denial of illness, awareness, preparation, rebuilding, and growth); this approach views everyone is "in recovery," regardless of their functioning and symptomatic expression (Andresen, Oades, & Caputi, 2003). Both definitions of recovery emphasize the importance of self-determination or self-management, with hope being an essential motivator to help achieve a fulfilled life (Shepherd, Boardman, & Slade, 2008).

When considering these definitions, however, it is no wonder that mental health clinicians are somewhat at a loss regarding which interventions do or do not promote their clients' overall recovery. Noordsy and colleagues (2002) have operationalized some of the major criteria of recovery into workable units. Figure 2.3 shows some of the major elements of recovery mentioned in the consumer-survivor literature, such as finding hope in the future, taking personal responsibility for oneself, and getting on with life even with a mental illness. The figure also gives examples of some elements that might help achieve or work toward each recovery domain. As such, being able to manage one's illness leads one to take responsibility for one's life and not depend solely on others. These elements can enable clinicians, and clinical researchers, to offer and develop interventions that can help individuals with a specific recovery domain.

After having experienced psychosis, many will feel their sense of self is shattered and have difficulties foreseeing a positive future. Cognitive behavioral therapy for psychosis can integrate the recovery model by helping people recognize their strengths

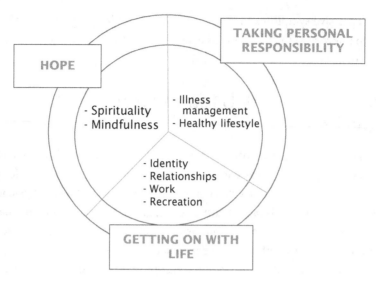

FIGURE 2.3 Recovery domains and intervention targets.

and positive qualities, accompanying them in setting and reaching their goals, as well as working together toward therapeutic goals that are important for the client first and foremost, even if it means not focusing on psychotic symptoms for some but on other thoughts or behaviors. Group CBT is a particularly good context in which to apply the recovery model because it involves working as a team, all the clients and the therapists together, in helping everyone meet their therapeutic goals.

Group CBT for psychosis can help with many of the elements mentioned in Figure 2.3. It helps people take *personal responsibility* by managing their illness, using many of the techniques group CBT for psychosis offers, namely, by modifying their dysfunctional beliefs and specific behaviors. To help people *get on with their lives*, group CBT for psychosis can also help them redefine their goals and work on their self-esteem and identity. Group CBT for psychosis, by offering concrete tools and a supportive and positive interpersonal experience, also helps people find *hope* in their future. In fact, the group CBT for psychosis intervention as presented here is very much goal oriented and therefore, through meeting goals, encourages feelings of accomplishment and hope.

The *vulnerability-stress-competence* model is also quite useful in group CBT for psychosis. It is essentially a modified stress-diathesis model, described earlier to explain how schizophrenia evolves through the interaction of biological vulnerabilities and environmental stressors. The model was modified in 1982 by Liberman (Liberman, 1982) to include the elements of competence and protective factors, thereby giving back power to the individual regarding the course of his or her symptoms. As is reflected in Figure 2.4, individuals have various biological, genetic, or neurological vulnerabilities that can lead to psychotic symptoms when stressors, such as trauma, substance abuse, or constant daily stressors (bullying, racism), are present. However, someone who has strong family and social support, good communication skills in asking for help when needed, good

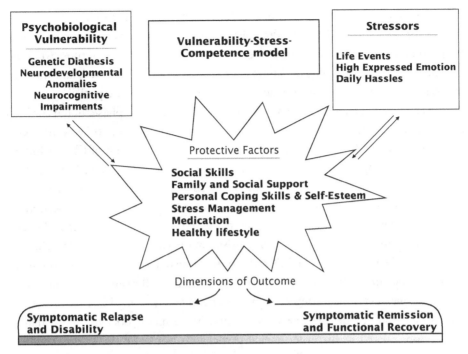

FIGURE 2.4 Vulnerability-stress-competence model.

self-esteem, good stress-management strategies, and a large and efficacious inventory of coping strategies when symptoms arise, and who responds well to his or her medication is much less likely to experience a symptomatic relapse when faced with stressors. These protective factors are all modifiable elements that can be learned, developed, and worked on. Group CBT for psychosis actually covers many of these protective factors, empowering individuals to feel they can have some control over their symptoms, instead of being passive victims of a brain disease—which, unfortunately, is a common message given by many mental health professionals. In fact, clinicians need to work with the person in improving or developing more and better protective factors. The vulnerability-stress-competence model has the advantage that it can be personalized, with each person recognizing his or her own vulnerabilities, stressors, and protective factors, realizing which of the latter need to be worked on and which are already quite well established.

Although the following models are not used to explain symptoms or behaviors, they are essential models in group psychotherapy for people with psychosis: the single-session frame model and the social learning model.

The *single-session model* essentially means that although group CBT happens over many sessions (typically between 16 and 24), each session must exist as an independent entity. It is clearly recognized that group process evolves over time, with increased feelings of cohesion (this will be discussed further in Chapter 4), and that learning in group CBT is incremental, with each session having a clear goal and offering a unique experience. There are multiple reasons for this. First, people with psychosis often have cognitive difficulties, such as with memory and attention, and having themes that cover more than one session will demand from the therapist a lot of repetition of what happened during the previous session. Second, there is a sense of accomplishment and purpose when each session is clearly defined. Clients know what they learned and covered, and they leave the session with a concrete experience in mind. Third, CBT and especially group CBT sessions involve a set agenda with a beginning, middle, and end phase. In the context of group CBT, the content of the sessions is typically planned ahead of time, while keeping in mind incremental learning, group process, and the introduction of CBT techniques. This step-by-step approach to learning, in which easy-to-understand and more basic concepts are introduced first, with more complex links brought later, helps motivate clients to attend sessions and also makes catching up easier for those who miss a session. The attention to group process means that activities with more difficult content or those that necessitate more sensitive self-disclosure arise only when strong group cohesion is in place. As for the introduction to CBT techniques, those that help create cohesion, such as normalization, are explained and used first, with more self-threatening techniques such as considering alternative beliefs brought in later. In emphasizing incremental learning, we wish to make it clear that the single-session frame model does not imply that sessions can be offered in any order or that participants can begin the group at any stage (see Chapter 6). It does mean that time management is crucial, that each session has a purpose, and that a session is a unique experience happening in the context of a theme, within a phase of the therapy.

Bandura's *social learning theory* (Bandura, 1977) stipulates that people learn better in a social context through modeling and observations. In group CBT for psychosis, learning is facilitated by the context, that is, people with similar issues. Modeling naturally occurs in a group setting with other participants, who are respected and valued once group cohesion is established, becoming models for their peers. Observational learning also occurs by seeing how the therapists work together (in co-therapy) and how other participants help each other in offering solutions, feedback, or ways of coping. Unlike some psychodynamic group psychotherapies that try to give the group a single voice, interpreting interactions (such as the Tavistock method [Semmelhack, Ende, & Hazell, 2013]), or that focus on each person individually (similar to a succession of brief individual therapies), each person is heard in group CBT for psychosis, with the others being active participants sharing their own experiences and offering feedback. Yet no participant is singled out because everyone works on his or her own issues linked to the common theme. Learning from each other, sharing similar experiences, and discovering new techniques and strategies together with the therapists are all central aspects of group CBT for psychosis.

Conclusion

Group CBT for psychosis not only was developed from individual CBT for psychosis, stemming mostly from studies on cognitive biases in psychosis and from cognitive theories of CBT for other disorders, but also integrates theories from psychiatric rehabilitation, such as the vulnerability-stress-competence model and the recovery model, while also considering essential group learning theories, such as Bandura's social learning theory and the single-session model. The integration of theories and concepts presented here is meant to offer an understanding of the influences behind the development of the group CBT for psychosis intervention. Of course, there are other influences, such as the developers' personal views on group psychotherapy and their own clinical experience, but here we have presented the essential empirical and theoretical influences behind the intervention that will be presented in detail in Chapters 6 to 10.

What Have Studies Taught Us About CBT for Psychosis?

Studies on CBT for psychosis have been ongoing since the early 1990s and have followed the traditional steps of psychotherapy research, whereby we find initial feasibility studies with no or poor control groups; larger, carefully controlled trials focusing on specific populations (high-risk, early psychosis, older participants, treatment resistant) or on symptoms or models; process-oriented studies; and integrative studies looking at CBT merged with other therapeutic models.

Initial Studies: Treatment-Resistant Psychosis

When looking back at initial studies, it is important to consider the context in which they were carried out. In the United Kingdom in the early 1990s, many creative psychologists were working in schizophrenia research looking into cognitive biases, developing detailed scales to assess psychotic symptoms, and applying this knowledge to tailoring CBT to help those with persistent psychotic symptoms (Tarrier et al., 1993; Chadwick & Lowe, 1990). Few, if any, psychological interventions were being offered to people with psychosis in the United Kingdom at the time, given that the leading psychiatric model was that schizophrenia was a brain disease. Therefore, the first studies on CBT for psychosis aimed at helping those who did not respond optimally to medication; these studies presented CBT for psychosis as an adjunctive treatment to medication, focusing mostly on psychotic symptoms. As Birchwood and Trower (2006) describe, this was a mistake that has stuck with the field for many years, since CBT for psychosis is not a pseudo-neuroleptic and does not solely aim at curing positive symptoms. In fact, CBT for psychosis might be more useful in helping people with the emotions linked to the psychotic experience, alleviating distress and improving self-esteem, for instance. Yet most of the early studies on CBT for psychosis were conducted with this "treatment-resistant" group of individuals and obtained highly significant clinical (and statistical) improvements in positive symptoms for those receiving the therapy compared with a treatment-as-usual group (Drury, Birchwood, Cochrane, & Macmillan, 1996; Kuipers et al., 1997; Tarrier et al., 1998).

The following studies involved more sophisticated trials, with carefully observed randomizations and at least some form of assessor blindness, and most also found significant advantages for the CBT for psychosis condition over the control condition, especially when the control condition was treatment as usual and not another treatment comparison. As mentioned by Wykes and colleagues (2008), as the quality of the trials improved, the effect sizes became somewhat smaller. This fact has been greatly criticized by biological psychiatrists who are campaigning against the use of CBT for psychosis (Lynch, Laws, & McKenna, 2010), but it is in fact a typical phenomenon found not only in psychotherapy research for other disorders (Wampold et al., 1997) but also in medication trials (Leucht et al., 2013). Indeed, even the best antipsychotics (e.g., clozapine) show only small effect sizes when compared with other antipsychotics. In fact, the artificial context of the trial results in the overall group showing smaller effect sizes than what can be found in more ecological studies (i.e., in the real world). In studies, CBT for psychosis (especially individual CBT for psychosis) typically does not show a large advantage over other psychological treatments such as supportive therapy or skills training, especially immediately following treatment. It is also important to mention that the control conditions used, at times real behavioral therapies focusing on problem-solving (Tarrier et al., 1993) or skills training (Lecomte et al., 2008) and at other times caring and positive conversations in a befriending context (Sensky et al., 2000), are meant to have some therapeutic effects. The effects were hypothesized as being not as important, not as specific, or not as long-lasting. Essentially, the studies on individuals with medication-resistant psychosis found that CBT for psychosis helped decrease psychotic symptoms at post-treatment, although rarely significantly more than control treatments, but that at follow-up the effects were typically maintained or greater compared with the control condition. Unfortunately, these first studies did not look at other variables that could have changed with CBT for psychosis, and none offered CBT for psychosis in a group context, except for a study by Wykes and colleagues (Wykes, Parr, & Landau, 1999) on voices that obtained improvements for part of the sample on diminishing hallucinations and improving functioning. It is also important to mention that many of the control treatments offered are seldom available in clinical settings. It is understandable that some stakeholders might consider it more cost-effective to offer supportive therapy or befriending rather than CBT for psychosis in their setting, but one should remember that these former treatments do not offer lasting effects, and CBT for psychosis does not have to be costly. In fact, when offered in groups and with regular mental health clinicians, it can be very cost-effective. More recently, a meta-analysis by Turner, van der Gaag, Kariotaki, and Cuijpers (2014) found stronger effects of CBT for psychosis on positive symptoms than for other psychological interventions (including befriending and supportive therapy), whereas skills training obtained better results on negative symptoms. Another recent meta-analysis on studies with people with medication-resistant psychosis describes that CBT for psychosis helps decrease psychotic and overall symptoms at posttreatment (medium effect size, Hedges's $g = 0.47$) and that the impact on symptoms is maintained at follow-up ($g = 0.41$; Burns, Erickson, & Brenner, 2014). Cognitive behavioral therapy for psychosis is now accepted around the world as an evidence-based treatment that should be offered to individuals with a diagnosis of schizophrenia who demand it, who experience distress linked to their symptoms, or who experience psychotic symptoms even though they receive antipsychotic medication (see, e.g., the National Institute for Health and Care Excellence [NICE] guidelines in the United Kingdom [NICE, 2009] or the Patient Outcomes Research Team [PORT] guidelines in the United States [Dixon et al., 2010]).

Studies on Specific Populations, Symptoms, or Models

The positive results obtained with persons who typically had been presenting with psychotic symptoms for many years created enthusiasm and brought clinical researchers to apply CBT for psychosis to different populations. The various populations targeted were linked to a stage of the illness (high-risk, early psychosis, relapse, medication refusers, older, and less symptomatic), were from specific cultural groups, or exhibited specific symptoms (voices [or even more specifically command hallucinations], paranoia, worry, and negative symptoms).

Specific Populations

The first high-risk study using CBT was conducted by Morrison and colleagues (2004), which involved offering CBT to young people who were considered at risk for developing psychosis because they had transient psychotic symptoms (brief limited intermittent psychotic symptoms) or attenuated (subclinical) psychotic symptoms, as well as a drop in functioning, some genetic or family predisposition to developing psychosis, or a diagnosis of schizotypal personality disorder. The individual CBT intervention that was offered did not necessarily target psychotic symptoms but had the aim of providing a more general set of skills that the young individuals could use when confronted with difficulties or stress. The first trial found very strong results for the intervention, with much lower rates of transition to psychosis than among those not who did not receive the intervention, but it presented with methodology flaws (i.e., randomization was not done effectively). The second trial (a larger, multisite trial, with a strict protocol) did not obtain the desired effects on the main outcome—in fact, the transition rates were fairly low for both conditions—but it did find some advantages for the CBT condition on secondary outcomes (Morrison et al., 2012). Similarly, a trial by Addington and colleagues (2011) using the same CBT protocol found slightly more conversions in the control condition than the CBT condition but no other differences in outcomes between the high-risk individuals receiving CBT or supportive therapy, except for perhaps slightly faster improvements on attenuated positive symptoms in the CBT group.

Individuals following a first or second episode of psychosis became an interesting target for CBT researchers. The largest study was the Socrates study (Lewis et al., 2002), covering a large part of England, in which individual CBT for psychosis was offered soon after people were hospitalized, with the control group receiving a befriending intervention. No important differences between the groups were found, except perhaps for the CBT group improving slightly faster and maintaining their improvements longer than the control condition. In fact, most of the CBT for early psychosis studies offering individual CBT have obtained modest results at most (Jackson et al., 2001; Lewis et al., 2002; Gleeson et al., 2013), especially when the intervention was offered early during the hospitalization. Of the few studies that have found significant improvements, our group CBT for psychosis study appeared to have obtained the strongest results, demonstrating not only symptomatic improvements even higher than the control condition (skills training for symptom management) but also improvements in self-esteem, social support, and coping strategies (Lecomte et al., 2008; Lecomte, Leclerc, & Wykes, 2012; Lecomte, Leclerc, Wykes, & Lecomte, 2003), described in more detail later in this chapter in the section on group CBT for psychosis.

Gumley and colleagues (2003) conducted a trial in which they offered CBT for psychosis to individuals who were beginning to experience a psychotic relapse, with the aim of stopping or diminishing the length or intensity of the relapse. Almost half the number of participants who had received CBT, rather than treatment as usual, relapsed at 12 months (i.e., 13 in CBT vs. 25 in treatment as usual), and overall the CBT group improved more on symptoms and social functioning.

Recently, Morrison and colleagues (2014) proposed to offer CBT for psychosis to individuals with a diagnosis of schizophrenia who refuse to take medication. A total of 74 individuals were randomized to individual CBT for psychosis or treatment as usual. The results showed that CBT for psychosis significantly decreased symptoms (overall and positive) in those who received it and that CBT for psychosis could be a viable treatment option for individuals who refuse to take medication.

As for older individuals, Granholm and colleagues (2005) have demonstrated that symptomatic improvements are not as marked, given a mostly stable clinical picture, but that group CBT combined with active skills training can help improve social functioning, improve insight, and decrease negative symptoms. Others, namely, from the Beck Institute (Grant, Huh, Perivoliotis, Stolar, & Beck, 2012), have also found that combining skills training and cognitive behavior therapy for older low-functioning individuals could help improve their functioning and decrease negative symptoms.

Recently, Naeem and colleagues (2015) revealed the results of the first random-ized controlled trial using a culturally adapted version of CBT for people with psy-chosis living in Pakistan. A total of 116 participants received either six individual sessions and one family session of CBT or treatment as usual. Results revealed sig-nificant improvements on positive and negative symptoms compared with the control condition (Naeem et al., 2015). Other cultural adaptations are warranted to deter-mine whether CBT for psychosis is efficacious in non-Western countries other than Pakistan.

Specific Symptoms (Voices, Paranoia, Worry, Negative Symptoms)

Although most CBT for psychosis interventions are quite general and focus mostly on positive symptoms such as delusions and hallucinations, some are very specific in terms of the targeted symptom. One of these outcomes is voices. As mentioned previously, Til Wykes was the first to offer CBT for voices (Wykes et al., 2005), mostly looking at the presence or absence of hallucinations. Other studies have also shown interest in CBT for voices, such as ones by Mark van der Gaag and colleagues (2012) focusing on diminish-ing the distress associated with the perceived power of the voice, and by Max Birchwood and colleagues (2011) using CBT for psychosis strategies to diminish threatening voices, namely, command hallucinations, looking at changes in the frequency of the voices but also in the interpretation of the voice's power and knowledge (omnipotence and omni-science) and the changes in the voice hearer's behaviors linked to the voice (compliance or resistance). A preliminary trial (Trower et al., 2004) did find that CBT for psychosis helped decrease compliance behaviors (i.e., doing what the voice commands) and beliefs linked to the voices, as well as diminish depression and distress, but not frequency or attributes of the voices. A recent pilot study described a web-based CBT for psychosis intervention for voices (Gottlieb, Romeo, Penn, Mueser, & Chiko, 2013) with similar sig-nificant results.

Although many pilot studies targeting persecutory delusions have been published, Freeman and colleagues (2015) are the first to publish the results of a large randomized controlled trial ($N = 150$) specifically targeting worry and paranoid delusions. The results strongly favor the six-session CBT intervention with significant reductions in worry and persecutory delusions.

Another symptom that has been targeted in CBT for psychosis is negative symp-toms. Very few trials have been specifically designed to offer CBT for negative symp-toms alone. As such, Staring and colleagues (2013) have presented pilot data suggesting promising improvements in negative symptoms. However, the TONES study (Klingberg et al., 2011), a larger trial, did not find any advantage of CBT over cognitive remedia-tion therapy for cognitive deficits (memory or attention) in terms of improving negative symptoms and even found that some had gotten worse.

Meta-analyses

At the time this chapter was written, 20 meta-analyses pertaining to the efficacy or effectiveness of CBT for psychosis had been published, covering a total of more than 40 randomized controlled trials. The major ones are described in Table 3.1 (Gould, Mueser, Bolton, Mays, & Goff, 2001; Pilling et al., 2002; Zimmermann, Favrod, Trieu, & Pomini,

TABLE 3.1 Selection of meta-analyses on CBT for psychosis

Authors (Year)	Scope of Meta-analysis	Number of Studies in Meta-analysis	Conclusions
Gould et al. (2001)	All controlled studies on CBT for psychosis	7 (N = 340)	Post-therapy mean effect sizes were moderate (0.65), with large follow-up effects (0.93).
Pilling et al. (2002)	All RCTs using CBT for psychosis	8 (N = 393)	Important improvements in mental state maintained at follow-up. Lower dropout rates for CBT.
Zimmerman et al. (2005)	All controlled studies on CBT for psychosis	14 (N = 1,484)	Significant improvements in positive symptoms. Bigger effect sizes for acute (0.57) compared with chronic condition (0.27).
Wykes et al. (2008)	All published studies on CBT for psychosis	34 (N = 1,964)	CBT for psychosis offers moderate effect sizes (0.4) on symptoms (general and positive). Effect sizes are bigger for less rigorous studies.
Granhom et al. (2009)	All published CBT for psychosis measuring social functioning	18 (N = 1,378)	CBT for psychosis improves social functioning in two thirds of studies; the other one third only improved in symptoms.
Álvarez-Jiménez et al. (2011)	All psychosocial and pharmacological treatments for relapse in early psychosis	3 individual CBT for psychosis (N = 283)	No advantage of CBT for psychosis over specialized first-episode treatment.
Sarin et al. (2011)	All controlled CBT for psychosis studies with low risk of bias	22 (N = 2,469)	Trend favoring CBT for psychosis at post-treatment. Strong evidence for CBT for psychosis over other treatments at follow-up (small effect size).
Hofman et al. (2012)	All published CBT for all psychological problems	18 meta-analyses/ reviews for psychosis	CBT for psychosis shows small to medium effect sizes for positive and negative symptoms, medium effect sizes for secondary outcomes (functioning, mood, social anxiety).
Hutton & Taylor (2013)	CBT for psychosis for high risk	6 (N = 800)	CBT reduces by at least 50% rate of transition to psychosis compared with control condition. Reduced symptoms only at 12 months, and no apparent impact on functioning.
Turner et al. (2014)	Psychological interventions for psychosis	48 (N = 3,295)	CBT for psychosis is more effective than all other interventions (pooled) in reducing positive symptoms. Skills training shows stronger effects for improving negative symptoms.

2005; Wykes, Steel, Everitt, & Tarrier, 2008; Hofmann, Asnaani, Vonk, Sawyer, & Fang, 2012; Sarin, Wallin, & Widerlöv, 2011; Turner et al., 2014), along with their main conclusions. Some other meta-analyses (not included in the table) present a clear bias against CBT for psychosis (e.g., Lynch et al., 2010; Jauhar et al., 2014), trying to demonstrate that the small effect sizes they find justify eliminating CBT for psychosis from national guidelines such as NICE (NICE, 2009) or PORT (Dixon et al., 2010). Given that they present the only meta-analyses not favoring CBT for psychosis and that they have excluded several studies from their meta-analyses, their conclusions need to be taken lightly. As described earlier, as the studies become more sophisticated and rigorous, comparing CBT for psychosis to other active treatments, the meta-analyses describe more modest effect sizes (Wykes et al., 2008). Many of the more recent meta-analyses tend to focus on specific symptoms or variables, such as improvement in social functioning (Granholm, Ben-Zeev, & Link, 2009), or on targeted clienteles (early psychosis [Álvarez-Jiménez, Parker, Hetrick, McGorry, & Gleeson, 2011] or prodromal/at risk for psychosis [Hutton & Taylor, 2013]). Although CBT for psychosis is offered in many modalities, by therapists of different levels of competence and using different techniques or philosophies, most meta-analyses support the use of CBT for psychosis for improving symptoms, decreasing distress, and improving other indices of well-being such as social functioning, self-esteem, and quality of life, often with larger effect sizes at follow-up than immediately after treatment, suggesting sustained gains. Only a small number of the studies included in the meta-analyses used a group CBT for psychosis format.

Group CBT for Psychosis

Fewer studies have investigated the effects of group CBT for psychosis than of individual CBT for psychosis. In the 1990s only a few studies investigated groups: two from our team using the cognitive and behavioral model, as well as other models, to improve the self-esteem (Lecomte et al., 1999) and strategies for coping with stress (Leclerc, Lesage, Ricard, Lecomte, & Cyr, 2000) of people with chronic schizophrenia. Although these groups are not pure CBT for psychosis, and are presented in more detail in Chapter 14, they obtained significant results in terms of diminishing positive symptoms of psychosis and improving self-esteem, coping strategies, and functioning (Table 3.2). Wykes and colleagues (1999), the other pioneers in group CBT for psychosis, developed a brief group therapy for people struggling with voices and obtained promising results. Other groups, combining CBT for psychosis with social skills training, for instance (Granholm et al., 2005), or offering CBT for psychosis in a brief group format for inpatients (Owen et al., 2015), also obtained positive results. Most groups follow a typical group therapy model (explained in Chapter 4), except for Granholm's group, which is slightly different (open group, with modules repeated). Only two group studies did not obtain strong results. The first, by Barrowclough et al. (2006), appears to have essentially transposed individual CBT for psychosis to a group format with no detailed information regarding training in

TABLE 3.2 Studies on group CBT for psychosis

Authors (Year)	Design	Aim	Outcomes
Lecomte et al. (1999)	RCT (exp. vs. TAU), 24 group sessions (N = 95)	Improve self-esteem (Reasoner's developmental model)	Improved positive symptoms and coping strategies for experimental group
Wykes et al. (1999)	Pilot study, 6 group sessions (N = 21)	Coping with voices (cognitive strategies)	Diminished perception of voice power, diminished distress, improved coping
Leclerc et al. (2000)	RCT (exp. vs. TAU), 24 group sessions (N = 99)	Improve stress management (Lazarus's model)	Improved positive symptoms, self-esteem and hygiene for experimental group
Chadwick et al. (2000)	Pilot study, 8 group sessions (N = 22)	Diminish distress with voices	Diminished power of voice and feelings of control by voice
Granholm et al. (2005)	RCT (exp. vs. TAU), 24 sessions (N = 76)	Combined CBT and social skills training to improve functioning in older patients	No effects on symptoms; improved functioning, improved coping and insight for experimental group
Wykes et al. (2005)	RCT (exp. vs. TAU), 7 sessions (N = 85)	Improve coping with voices and functioning	Effects on hallucinations only in the experimental groups with more expert therapists; improvements in social functioning (experimental only)
Barrowclough et al. (2006)	RCT (exp. vs. TAU), 18 sessions (N = 113)	Improve positive symptoms	No effects on symptoms; improvements only on hopelessness and self-esteem
Landa et al. (2006)	Pilot study, 13 group sessions (N = 6)	Improve paranoia (CBT for psychosis)	Diminished conviction in paranoid delusion, diminished distress
McLeod et al. (2007)	Small RCT (exp. vs. TAU) 8 group sessions (N = 20)	Diminish voices, improve coping with voices (CBT)	Diminished frequency and power of voices for experimental group
Lecomte et al. (2008)	RCT (exp. vs. skills training vs. TAU), 24 group sessions (N = 129)	Improve symptoms and distress in early psychosis (CBT for psychosis)	Improved positive symptoms (both treatments), improved negative and overall symptoms (experimental only); improved self-esteem, coping skills, and social support (experimental only)
Penn et al. (2009)	RCT (exp. vs. supportive therapy), 12 group sessions (N = 65)	Coping with voices (Wykes's module—cognitive strategies)	Better at resisting voices, perceived less power in voices, more improvements in overall symptoms for experimental group
Borras et al. (2009)	RCT (exp. vs. TAU), 24 sessions (N = 54)	Improve self-esteem (Lecomte's module)	Improved self-esteem, assertiveness, coping strategies and symptoms for experimental group (more for those with staff support)
Raune & Law (2013)	Pilot study, varying session lengths, various client profiles (N = 58)	Diminish symptoms using modular symptom-specific CBT groups (each small module = new group, different participants and therapists)	Poor attendance; no clear benefits
Owen et al. (2015)	Quasi experimental (exp. vs. TA), 4 inpatient CBT for psychosis group sessions (N = 113)	Reduce distress, improve confidence and diminish positive symptoms.	Decrease in distress and improved confidence in dealing with one's mental health in the CBT for psychosis group only

group therapy or recognition of group processes presented in the article, suggesting that the absence of results might be linked to these two factors (this is only a hypothesis). The second, by Raune and Shaw (2013), did not follow basic rules of group therapy and changed participants and therapists for each small module, never really enabling a sense of cohesion (essential elements of group therapy will be discussed in Chapter 4).

As for our own group CBT for psychosis, explained in detail in this book, we conducted a large randomized controlled trial over 5 years with individuals presenting with early psychosis (see Lecomte et al., 2008). Although the study was conducted with early psychosis, the group module has since been used with individuals with a longer course of illness with similar results reported (not published). In fact, the module is currently being used in more than 13 countries.

Our trial aimed at adapting CBT for psychosis to be more accessible to those needing it by offering a structured module that all could follow (therapists and participants), giving the therapy in a group context (therefore enabling more participants to receive the intervention at the same time), and having the intervention delivered by mental health workers with an understanding of CBT for psychosis but with very little CBT for psychosis training—in fact, having received only 2 days of intensive training. To ensure continued use of the therapy after the trial was over, the groups were delivered by at least one mental health worker from the clinic where the participants were recruited. We also aimed at determining not only if our group CBT for psychosis would offer similar results as other studies using individual CBT for psychosis, but also if it would be any better than an already existing evidence-based treatment, namely, skills training for symptom management. This latter intervention (see Chapter 1 for more details on skills training) was also offered in group format and helped participants recognize their symptoms, the warning signs that indicate they may be close to a relapse, how to use various coping strategies, and how to discuss important symptom-related issues with mental health workers. The essence of the intervention, namely, symptoms, was very similar to that of the CBT for psychosis module except it was tackled in a very different manner, using more behavioral strategies, more psychoeducation, and no attempts to actually try to change the beliefs linked to the symptoms. We felt it would be a good comparison group, and in fact it was.

The results of our study, described in greater detail by Lecomte et al. (2008) and Lecomte et al. (2012), showed that, compared with the wait-list control group, participants who received both treatments greatly improved in positive symptoms of psychosis at post-treatment and at 6-month follow-up. Only the CBT for psychosis group showed significant improvements on general symptoms over time, as well as on negative symptoms. It also appeared that group CBT for psychosis was preferred by many, given the higher retention rate in the groups and in the study compared with the skills training approach. Another interesting result pertained to psychosocial variables, which had been scarcely looked at in most CBT for psychosis studies at the time. Individuals in the group CBT for psychosis, but not in the other conditions, improved on self-esteem and on coping skills during the course of the treatment, feeling more confident in themselves and using more active coping strategies when confronted with stress. They also improved at 6-month follow-up on social support, particularly attachment with others. This result was further investigated at the 1-year follow-up (for those we were able to assess), and it seemed that group CBT for psychosis had a continued impact on social support, with participants becoming even better at developing supportive relationships. Although this might appear strange, such improved social support over time has been reported in other studies using group approaches for other conditions, such as complicated grief (Ogrodniczuk, Joyce, & Piper, 2003); it appears that the social context of the group helps people acquire the needed skills to continue developing a support network outside the group and after the therapy has ended. Furthermore, changes in beliefs were maintained at 1 year post-treatment (Lecomte et al., 2012), although some symptoms appeared to fluctuate, that is, people were no longer convinced of the reality of their delusions or the power of their voices, even if they still could hear voices or at times have unusual thoughts. It appears that for early psychosis at least, the group format is more effective, even if it is delivered by nonexpert CBT therapists (Saksa, Cohen, Srihari, & Woods, 2009).

Process-Oriented Studies

Now that the scientific and clinical communities have essentially accepted that CBT for psychosis is a noteworthy treatment with multiple potential benefits to those who receive it, researchers are interested in understanding in more detail what makes it work, and for whom. The processes involved and the essential ingredients that make CBT for psychosis work are still being investigated, although some results have emerged, namely, regarding aspects of the therapy, client characteristics, relationship aspects between the client and therapist, and characteristics of the therapists.

Aspects of the Therapy

It is difficult to determine exactly which techniques or aspects of CBT for psychosis are essential. Morrison and Barratt (2010) have conducted a Delphi study that involved asking several expert CBT for psychosis therapists what they would consider the essential elements of CBT for psychosis, and these therapists rated 77 elements as extremely important. Some of these elements involved attitudes and relational aspects, as well as specific techniques. A recent study looking at the most active ingredients in CBT for psychosis for individuals considered at high risk to develop psychosis suggests that the use of a CBT formulation and of regular homework improved the outcomes (Flach et al., 2015). There is currently no consensus in the field regarding whether CBT for psychosis absolutely needs an individual formulation of the person's problems or whether a more generic model, used in a manualized treatment, for instance, is good enough. Homework is, however, mentioned by many as being an important ingredient (Morrison & Barratt, 2010). It is also important to realize that there is no "one size fits all" for CBT for psychosis, even when using a manualized approach. In fact, therapists will help clients focus more on specific aspects of their experience and might use more cognitive or more behavioral techniques depending on the person's profile and comprehension of the therapy. A recent qualitative study (Berry & Hayward, 2011) looking at nine clients' experience of CBT for psychosis and what they considered the essential elements revealed that specific techniques and principles of CBT for psychosis, such as normalization and seeking facts or alternative explanations, were seen as very helpful. Another study (G. Dunn et al., 2012) found that although they could not pinpoint which specific techniques were essential, clients who received only partial therapy involving only the engagement part, did not benefit as much as those who received the complete treatment. The researchers concluded that the number of sessions of CBT for psychosis received was linked to clinical outcomes. This result can be interpreted both as a dose effect, whereby the more CBT for psychosis you receive, the more likely you will benefit from the experience, and as a sign that some people might need longer treatment or more sessions of CBT for psychosis.

Client Characteristics

Is CBT for psychosis meant for everyone, or do some clients benefit more than others? This question has not yet been answered, but researchers have found some interesting results. Cognitive flexibility prior to receiving CBT for psychosis, that is, being open to considering alternatives for beliefs, was found by some to predict better outcomes (Garety et al., 1997; Brabban, Tai, & Turkington, 2009; Naeem, Kingdon, & Turkington, 2008). Others have found that subjects' having some form of insight into their illness (Naeem et al., 2008), believing they had some responsibility (personal attribution) regarding the cause of the illness (Freeman et al., 2013), thinking they are responsible for change in their lives (Myhr et al., 2013), and feeling optimistic about the future also predicted better outcomes. Essentially, CBT for psychosis works mostly for those who are willing and open to see things differently and wish to change. Other attributes have also been reported, namely, being female (Brabban et al., 2009), presenting with fewer negative symptoms (such as lack of motivation, lack of emotional expression, lack of pleasure; Thomas, Rossell, Farhall, Shawyer, & Castle, 2011), and having higher social functioning before therapy (Allott et al., 2011). Personality traits, specifically conscientiousness—meaning to act efficiently with self-discipline and planning ahead—have also been linked to greater outcomes in group CBT for psychosis (Beauchamp, Lecomte, Lecomte, Leclerc, & Corbière, 2013), especially regarding increased use of active coping strategies to deal with stress. None of these results have been replicated, and they should therefore be considered with caution. In fact, most CBT for psychosis therapists would say that CBT for psychosis should be offered to all who are experiencing distress and who demonstrate an interest in receiving it given that we cannot predict who will or will not benefit from it. It is always possible to present concepts in simpler or more complex terms, or to suggest more cognitive or behavioral strategies, depending on the clients' strengths and weaknesses.

Client-Therapist Relationship

In discussions of the relationship between the client and the therapist, studies most often refer to it as the *alliance*. The alliance measures how well the client and therapist agree on what is important in terms of goals and tasks, as well as the trusting bond they have developed together. The importance of the alliance as linked to clinical outcomes is more and more evident in CBT for psychosis studies. Studies in CBT for psychosis have demonstrated links between the strength of the therapeutic alliance and symptom reduction (Lecomte, Laferriere-Simarc, & Leclerc, 2011), higher attendance and participation in CBT for psychosis (Bentall et al., 2002; Johnson, Penn, Bauer, Meyer, & Evans, 2008; Lecomte et al., 2011), and increased self-esteem (Lecomte et al., 2011). A study by Hazel Dunn and colleagues (2006) found that a stronger alliance was linked to better completion of homework assignments in CBT for psychosis. Fluctuations in the alliance as assessed by the client have been found to be linked to worse negative symptoms at post-therapy (Lecomte et al., 2011). Group cohesion, essentially the alliance between all members in a group, is also considered a strong predictor of therapeutic outcomes (Joyce, Piper, & Ogrodniczuk, 2007). Even though the alliance is considered essential to CBT for psychosis, there is still a paucity of studies that have looked closely at the alliance or group cohesion in connection with stages of the therapy or clinical outcomes.

A recent study by our team has found that the alliance and group cohesion are not stable phenomena in group CBT for psychosis and that they are particularly influential at key moments in the therapy, such as when alternative explanations for beliefs are being explored or new coping strategies are being tried. Aspects of group cohesion such as "personal compatibility" and "perceiving positive qualities in others" (other participants in the group and the therapists) are some of the strongest predictors, along with the alliance with the therapist, of improvements following CBT for psychosis (Lecomte, Leclerc, Wykes, Nicole, & Baki, 2014). Although we will describe the importance of these factors in more detail in the next chapter, it is noteworthy that these relational therapeutic factors are not solely theoretically based but have been proven in studies, such as the ones just described.

Therapist Characteristics

What do we know regarding therapist characteristics in CBT for psychosis? Not much, really. Few studies have looked at specific therapist characteristics, other than trying to determine if expert therapists are needed and if they need to be psychologists. Studies have found that clinicians from fields other than psychology, namely, psychiatrists, psychiatric nurses (Durham et al., 2003), occupational therapists, or social workers (Lecomte et al., 2008), could offer CBT for psychosis effectively with appropriate training. What is appropriate training is another issue and varies according to authors and according to the use or not of a structured manual. For instance, in our trial on group CBT for psychosis compared with group skills training, the therapists were expert mental health clinicians but not expert CBT for psychosis therapists. They all received a 2-day intensive training with role plays, followed a structured manual, and were supervised weekly. On average, the therapists did what was expected of them and received a fidelity score of 73% on the group-modified version of the Cognitive Therapy Scale (Young & Beck, 1980), meaning that they were conducting CBT for psychosis with some areas needing improvement (mostly clearly stating the agenda and encouraging homework). Kråkvik and colleagues (2013) also found that nonexperts could deliver quality CBT for psychosis. Although these studies did not find a link between therapist expertise and outcomes, others have suggested such a link (Wykes et al., 2005). Most studies, however, have looked at fidelity scores, meaning whether the therapists actually did what they were supposed to, but none looked at competency (i.e., how well they were actually doing it). There is a dearth of studies on the link between actual therapist competency and outcomes in CBT for psychosis. Similarly, little is known regarding what it really takes to be a competent CBT for psychosis therapist. Although we explore this question in more detail in Chapter 13, it is important to keep in mind that from the clients' perspective, a competent therapist is considered an essential element (Lecomte et al., 2012), although what they mean by it is not clear either. More studies are warranted to better define the necessary qualities, attitudes, and characteristics of CBT for psychosis therapists, not only to better understand the links with outcomes but also to improve the training currently offered to CBT for psychosis therapists.

Integrated Treatment Studies

Integrated treatments can be defined in many ways. One can integrate elements from different schools of thought, merge two psychotherapies or a psychotherapy with another form of treatment, or offer a therapy framework that can be applied within various therapeutic modalities, regardless of the school of thought. Some studies have investigated treatments integrating CBT for psychosis with some other treatment. We mentioned earlier a study by Granholm and colleagues (2005) in which skills training was added to CBT for psychosis and which obtained significant improvements on negative symptoms and functioning. Although some might consider skills training as part of CBT for psychosis, they are not traditionally offered together. Skills training is much more common in North America, where social skills training was a significant part of the deinstitutionalization movement as described in Chapter 1, than in European countries such as the United Kingdom. In fact, most CBT for psychosis offered in the United Kingdom, for instance, would be described as having more "cognitive" than "behavioral" components, whereas skills training is essentially behavioral. Other integrative approaches have been described but only as promising case studies. For instance, Hasson-Ohayon (2012) describes three case studies where CBT for psychosis and intersubjective therapy (an integrative approach in itself that uses a psychodynamic framework and humanistic techniques) were offered together. Some studies support integrating CBT for psychosis with third wave cognitive behavioral therapies (Chadwick, Hughes, Russell, Russell, & Dagnan, 2009), with family psychoeducation (Leclerc & Lecomte, 2012), or with supported employment (Lecomte, Corbière, & Lysaker, 2014; see Chapter 14). Lysaker and colleagues (Lysaker & Roe, 2012) have developed a metatheoretical approach to psychotherapy, involving focusing on metacognition (such as self and other appraisals of emotions and thoughts, and mastery in the face of adversity) using narratives that could be used within a CBT for psychosis framework. More studies are warranted, however, before suggesting that these novel integrative approaches are useful or efficacious.

Conclusion

Studies have shown that CBT for psychosis is an efficacious and effective treatment for people presenting with psychotic symptoms, distress, and other difficulties. Cognitive behavioral therapy for psychosis appears to help people at different stages of the illness, although some formats of the therapy (groups) appear preferable for individuals at different stages, particularly people with early psychosis, or individuals who are isolated or older. It appears that single-symptom focused CBT for psychosis also has benefits. More studies are needed to increase our understanding of the mechanisms at play and how change is brought about. More client characteristics and essential elements of the therapy, such as the alliance and group cohesion, need to be investigated. Furthermore, therapist competencies need to be better understood and measured. Including CBT for psychosis as part of integrated therapies is just beginning and has not yet been studied extensively.

Essential Elements
of Group Therapy

This chapter describes the unique elements of group therapy in general, as well as in group CBT for psychosis more specifically. Elements such as normalization of experience, socialization, social support, interpersonal learning, group cohesion, task focus, a safe and respectful environment, and a goal-oriented approach are described and illustrated. Also, the importance of using a single-session time frame and of ensuring an enjoyable group experience is put forward.

From Yalom to Group CBT for Psychosis

Irvin Yalom was one of the first clinicians to investigate the therapeutic elements that explain change experienced by participants in group psychotherapy. The essential elements he describes in the fifth edition of *The Theory and Practice of Group Psychotherapy* (Yalom & Leszcz, 2005) will be presented and explained or renamed according to CBT for psychosis terminology.

Instillation of hope: What Yalom describes as instillation of hope is what others would call *positive expectancy*, referring to the idea that people who agree to attend group therapy must somehow believe it can help them. In fact, those who truly believe the therapy will be worthless tend to not show up or drop out after one or two sessions. This hope is not specific to group therapy and can be found in connection with all psychotherapies. Recently, we conducted a study (Lecomte, Leclerc, Wykes, Nicole, & Abdel Baki, 2014) that suggested that even those who are initially less optimistic about their future can benefit from group CBT for psychosis–as long as they believe enough in the therapy's worth to continue attending. There are many ways to help instill hope or increase expectations before participants start a group. One way is to mention results from previous studies that suggest this treatment has helped others. Another is to have someone who has graduated and benefited from the group come and talk to future participants about his or her experience in the group. Most participants will find hope if the treatment appears to be tailored for them and answers a need. Presenting group CBT for psychosis as a means of coping with adversity and symptoms appeals to many. For the more pessimistic clients (or those with more negative symptoms who lack motivation), suggesting that they try attending the group for a few sessions and also mentioning that they can leave if they do not like it is helpful; they will at least make new friends.

Universality: Universality is probably one of the strongest therapeutic elements in group therapy for people with psychosis. It is described as the feeling of not being the only one with difficulties, not being alone, and being similar to others in some ways. In CBT for psychosis it is also called *normalization*. Although normalization is possible in individual CBT for psychosis by giving examples of other people who have experienced similar difficulties, in group CBT for psychosis it happens naturally. Simply learning that others have also experienced voices, or that others in the group also felt they had to accomplish a special mission or that they had special powers, helps participants feel less bizarre or "alienated" and enables them not only to share their experience but also to become more open to change. For normalization to really have an impact, there needs to be a planned time in the sessions, early on but not in the first few sessions, when this sharing of difficult and similar experiences takes place. Some clinicians might find it surprising that even participants who strongly believe they are Jesus Christ, for instance, are happy to learn that someone else has the same belief (we have never seen a rivalry in which one participant would argue with another regarding who was the real one). Even in groups where only some participants hear voices, the normalization activity for the other participants can be about having experienced something highly distressing, such as their first hospitalization. In fact, the horror and trauma linked to the first hospitalization are often discussed in the group, leading to an increased feeling of normalization, as well as shared empathy and—unfortunately, very often—shared outrage.

Imparting information: Yalom describes imparting information as the more didactic content that is being transmitted implicitly or explicitly in group therapy. In group CBT for psychosis, some explicit psychoeducation often takes place, where information is imparted regarding the impact of stress on symptoms, the A-B-C model of CBT, for instance, or why a specific technique is worth trying and how it works. Given that in group CBT for psychosis the therapists are seen not as experts but rather as collaborators, their knowledge is shared and becomes accessible to participants to use for themselves. In fact, once the knowledge is shared, participants will often refer back to it to help other participants during future sessions. Implicitly, participants learn to work in a group while following a set of predetermined rules; such learning can be transposed to the school or work setting, as well as more generally to functioning in the community.

Altruism: Yalom defines *altruism* as the fact that participants gain from helping others. In group CBT for psychosis, participants share not only difficult experiences but also new ways to cope with them or with symptoms. Participants are encouraged to support others in the group and to offer suggestions, explore beliefs, and share personal strategies. Typically, individuals with a psychotic disorder are "taken care of" and told what to do by professionals and are scarcely recognized for their own input and experience. In group CBT for psychosis, their personal experience is respected, and participants feel empowered by realizing that they can help others and that they have something worthy to share. An illustration of this is helpful.

After 14 sessions, a young man attending group CBT for psychosis came to the group with a bag in which the participant next to him could see there was a rope. The young man admitted he had planned to hang himself later that day. The other participants in the group spontaneously asked why, trying to explore if he had been experiencing stress, asked questions regarding his beliefs and emotions, and tried to understand the situation that led to this decision. Some participants mentioned alternatives to suicide, others tried to use cognitive dissonance to dissuade him ("I thought you believed in God. God doesn't want people to take their own lives"), and still others reminded him of his strengths and positive qualities and said that everyone in the group would miss him. Finally, participants discussed what had helped them at times when they were feeling despair, sharing the coping strategies they had used in the past to survive suicidal thoughts. Essentially, and without prompts, the participants used concepts and techniques they had learned so far in the group CBT for psychosis to help a fellow participant. And it worked—the participant completed the therapy and, when we last heard, was doing well.

The corrective recapitulation of the primary family group: Yalom believed that the group could replicate and repair family relationships. Although most therapists agree that past issues with one's parents and family can influence one's present behaviors and beliefs, in group CBT for psychosis the group is not considered a family but a group of close acquaintances or potential new friends. Given that therapists are not portraying themselves as experts or authority figures but instead participate in the group along with the other participants (while maintaining the structure and respecting the time frame), they are not perceived as parents but can be seen as models. When possible, we tend to recommend that co-therapists be of different genders, not because they represent parental figures but because some participants may find it more difficult to talk to a man or to a woman and also because it offers a model of good communication and collaboration between people of different genders. Given that groups will often include people of similar age (see Chapter 6), the group experience is not so much a corrective experience of the primary family as a positive experience of peer support.

Development of socializing techniques: People with psychotic disorders tend to isolate themselves, often initially because their symptoms create fear, misunderstanding, and a need to self-protect, and eventually because of broken ties with their network after their psychotic break or hospitalization. Social contacts can become feared in many ways: fear of acting strangely and being judged, fear of stigma toward people with mental illness, fear of not being interesting (or attractive) enough, or fear of not grasping the content of the social situation (e.g., not getting a joke). Furthermore, interactions with mental health professionals are rarely reciprocal and tend to encourage monologues about very personal aspects of one's life. Such interactions are not considered appropriate in the "real world." Groups are the perfect context for learning and practicing real-life interactions involving inquiring about the other, sharing, helping, and simply having conversations about leisure topics. In fact, group CBT for psychosis not only maximizes socialization during the sessions but also reserves a socialization and snack period at the end of each session for people who would like more time to chat and get to know each other. Contrary to other group approaches, group CBT for psychosis actually encourages friendships, and participants often socialize with other group members outside of the group, such as going out for coffee or taking part in other activities. The graduation party, after the last group session (described in more detail in Chapter 10), is also an important social event that the group organizes together.

Imitative behavior: In group therapy both the therapists and the group members can become models for the participants. Participants might be interested in trying a strategy or technique proposed by the therapist, but they might be even more willing to try a strategy proposed by another participant, whom they respect and identify with. A good example of this happened during a session in which we were discussing coping strategies to use when symptoms or stress become overwhelming. In addition to the long list that we give out, participants are encouraged to share their own strategies for others to try. One participant mentioned that what worked for her was taking a bath and playing with the faucets with her feet (opening the cold, then the hot, and so on). This seemed to the therapists a particularly funny, or odd, strategy. To our surprise, at the next session we learned that almost all the participants in the group had decided to try it and had found it very helpful! During the sessions, shy participants might become more assertive, imitating more outgoing participants, and participants who have refused to take their medication might become more adherent after hearing how medication helps others in the group. Given the influence the group has, the therapist's role is to ensure that positive imitation takes place and to steer the conversation away from negative coping strategies such as taking street drugs or resorting to violence.

Interpersonal learning: Yalom describes interpersonal learning as a complex interaction of human beings acting out their pathologies within the group; through interactions with the other participants and with insight and the therapist's input, participants learn to correct these emotional experiences. Group CBT for psychosis sees interpersonal learning very differently. For one thing, the groups are structured and do not allow (or encourage) re-enactment of negative interactions between group members. These would be seen as obstacles to the treatment. The group is, however, a perfect social context to help clients develop tolerance for others, reciprocity, and feelings of attachment, which have repercussions in their post-therapy lives. As mentioned in the previous chapter, social support—particularly attachment—not only improved during the group CBT for psychosis in our study but continued to improve in the 6 months and 1 year following the end of the group (Lecomte, Leclerc, & Wykes, 2012; Lecomte et al., 2008). This result suggests that the interpersonal learning that takes place within the group can be replicated outside, with other people, and leads to a strong social network.

Group cohesiveness: Group cohesion is probably the most recognized and most studied essential group psychotherapy element. In individual therapy, the alliance between the therapist and the client, namely, the development of a trusting bond, common goals, and agreed-upon tasks, has been found to moderate the effects of the therapy, suggesting that without a strong alliance people do not benefit as much from therapy (Castonguay, Constantino, & Holtforth, 2006). In group psychotherapy, the alliance becomes group cohesion. It does not, however, only involve agreeing on goals and tasks between the group members (including the therapists) but also implies the development of a gestalt. Indeed, the cohesion can be described as a sense of "wholeness" whereby participants feel they relate to each other, appreciate each other, and feel that they have things in common, and together have developed a group identity.

Cohesion does not always happen naturally in a group. Many factors can facilitate it, such as the choice of participants of similar ages or intellectual levels (see Chapter 6). Although sharing difficult experiences, such as in normalization activities, can help, sharing positive experiences helps as well. Sessions that aim at increasing one's self-esteem, exploring values, or sharing accomplishments and interests also help in building strong group cohesion. Sharing a common goal (e.g., coping with their symptoms) can bring people together as well. Typically, in our experience, strong group cohesion in individuals with psychosis (and who are still experiencing psychotic symptoms) takes about one month to build, when sessions are offered twice per week. However, some aspects of group cohesion, such as feeling compatible with others in the group and seeing positive qualities in the other group members, can happen very quickly (within three to four sessions) and often distinguish those who leave from those who remain in the group. The sooner participants feel they belong to the group, the more likely they will remain in the group until the last session.

Catharsis: In the fifth edition of *The Theory and Practice of Group Psychotherapy,* the therapeutic factor known as *catharsis* is treated along with other factors rather than considered a stand-alone factor as it was in previous editions. The concept of catharsis, or "getting things off one's chest," might not be therapeutic in itself unless it involves, as we propose for group CBT for psychosis, links with current thoughts, emotions, and behaviors. The act of sharing personal information, at times difficult information, is never imposed but can bring someone to see things differently, especially, as in group CBT for psychosis, when others offer their perspective (or alternative views) on the information shared. It can also lead to potential solutions regarding what can be achieved now, given this information. Unlike other therapies in which sharing personal information might be considered sufficient in itself, in group CBT for psychosis we do not let the person leave without feeling that this sharing has been useful or will be useful in a specific way (normalizing, for instance, or helping understand why the person has specific beliefs or helping others by offering one's own experience and coping strategies).

Other Therapeutic Factors Specific to Group CBT for Psychosis

Yalom's therapeutic factors are often general, and many can be applied to most psychotherapeutic groups, with clients presenting with various profiles or difficulties. Other therapeutic factors are essential when working with people with psychosis in particular and contribute to group CBT for psychosis's therapeutic effects.

Safe/respect: It may seem obvious that a group therapy should offer a safe environment where one can speak freely and not fear what will happen in the group. Yet, for individuals with paranoid features, making the group feel safe can be a challenge. There are some ways for therapists to make the group safe. The first is by offering a workbook covering the themes that will be discussed at each session within the group. This enables clients who are particularly worried and untrusting to feel safer, knowing that no surprise awaits them. Another is by setting rules from the start regarding respecting each other (i.e., that no negative comments, judgments, or ridicule of other participants is allowed in the group), which can also help instill a feeling of a safe haven. Finally, respecting people's pace can facilitate this feeling. For example, a man in one of our groups refused to share anything for more than a month (roughly eight sessions), although he regularly showed up and wrote in his workbook. After this time, he chose to actively participate in the group by sharing his thoughts, opinions, and difficulties. He admitted that it had taken him that long to make sure the group was safe and to ensure that no one hated him for having been particularly violent during his last psychosis-related hospitalization (some of the participants had been hospitalized at the same time as him). Respecting his pace enabled him to become an active member for the remainder of the sessions.

What happens when a group is not safe and respectful? A good example of this is portrayed in the film version of *One Flew Over the Cuckoo's Nest* (1975). Early on in the movie, the patients residing in the psychiatric institution (asylum) are told it is their group time. The nurse tries to get someone to initiate a group theme or discussion, but everyone seems anxious and unwilling to share anything. She then summarizes the last group session, which essentially dealt with a single participant's issues regarding his worries that his wife is having an extramarital affair, and then asks to continue on that topic. The participant is obviously uneasy and tries to justify his belief, in a defensive tone, using metaphors and a psychotic discourse. In response, other participants start making fun of him. The session turns into a screaming match, with the nurse calmly taking notes and once offering an interpretation. This scene clearly illustrates how the actions of an incompetent therapist, who does not provide a safe and structured setting and who chooses an inappropriate topic for discussion, can result in disrespectful interactions and a harmful group session.

Task focused: Group CBT for psychosis is extremely task focused in the sense that sessions have specific purposes that are translated into concrete discussion themes and active tasks during the sessions. Homework should not be the only "practice time" during group CBT for psychosis. In fact, each session is designed to have participants work on their issues, grasp new concepts, and discover new coping strategies by different means (e.g., working individually, in pairs, and everyone together). Being task focused does not mean that new issues cannot be addressed or that the workbook becomes an inflexible framework for each session. In fact, the task at hand might be for the group members to help a participant who is struggling on a particular day by using techniques and concepts they have learned. Being task focused means that everyone in the group knows what is being worked on and why, at each session. There is no "floating," with participants trying to find what to say; instead, there is a purpose to each session, and everyone knows what it is.

Goal oriented: In group CBT for psychosis, we utilize a goal-oriented approach, which flirts with positive psychology in many ways, focusing on strengths, goals, and positive qualities in order to empower the person facing adversities. People with psychosis are continually reminded of their difficulties by family members and clinicians, with symptoms and illness being part of the daily vocabulary, and strengths and goals scarcely spoken of. Experiences of stigma, of social isolation, and at times of feeling like a burden on their family can become overwhelming and result in forgetting that they are strong, capable people. By using a goal-oriented approach, participants in the group are considered first and foremost as people with potential, strengths, and positive qualities. This helps foster the self-confidence they need to believe they can achieve things in their lives and the belief that their "illness" will no longer determine who they are or what they can do. Of course, group CBT for psychosis deals with difficult thoughts and experiences, even suicidal thoughts, but we intentionally include sessions that boost self-esteem prior to discussing difficult themes and always make sure that even these difficult themes end on a positive note.

Out with the psychiatric vocabulary: There is a consensus among the CBT for psychosis scientific community and service user groups that labels such as diagnoses and psychiatric terms are not helpful for most clients. In group CBT for psychosis, we avoid using psychiatric diagnoses or naming symptoms at all. We believe that a participant does not need to admit to having a mental illness or to having experienced psychosis to take part in the group and that psychiatric terminology could in fact deter someone from attending. We do not speak of hallucinations, for instance, but mention voices or noises that others do not hear. Similarly, we do not mention delusions but instead describe unusual experiences or distressing thoughts. Of course, participants might wish to talk about their distressing thoughts of being lonely and not having friends, rather than the beliefs surrounding their recent psychotic episode. This would be fine, especially if making more friends was a goal. People with psychosis do not always mention psychotic symptoms as the most important thing to change in their lives when they start therapy. Many could in fact mention feelings of depression and sadness, or even feeling socially fearful, as being the most salient distress they are currently experiencing. By staying clear of psychiatric diagnoses and vocabulary, group CBT for psychosis also offers the chance for participants to use their own terms to describe their experiences. It helps participants to stop thinking about themselves and their situation through the psychiatric illness lens and to instead see themselves as individuals, not patients.

Single-session time frame: Several reasons justify offering sessions that could exist as separate entities, meaning that each session covers a specific theme and includes a beginning, middle, and end. For one, designing single-session time frames suggests that the content has been simplified enough for people to grasp the essential elements of the concept in one session. Many people struggling with psychosis have the added burden of experiencing cognitive difficulties, such as poor memory, attention, and reasoning. This single-session time frame ensures that everyone gets the most out of each session, even if some aspects of previous sessions might have been forgotten. Participants at times miss a session, but they can work on the material of the missed session in the workbook alone and re-enter the group at the following session, without feeling lost or having the impression that they are interrupting. Furthermore, participants realize that they are actually accomplishing something at every session. This realization not only helps in ensuring attendance but also empowers participants, who see that they are learning new concepts and skills at each session. In fact, each session ends with a wrap-up in which everyone takes the time to reflect on, and write down, what they learned and wish to remember for that session.

Homework: The word *homework* can elicit negative memories for some, especially for participants who struggled (or are still struggling) in school. Some authors prefer to call homework in CBT *home exercise* or *practical exercise*. Regardless of its name, homework is considered an essential therapeutic factor in group CBT for psychosis, helping participants bring home what was done during the session. In a group, an exercise might appear clear and easy, but once the participant is alone at home, replicating it can be experienced as more demanding, yet it is important because it can enable the person to experience the application of a technique or skill in his or her real life. Most homework assignments in group CBT for psychosis are used as integration exercises that replicate what was learned and experienced in the group by using real-life situations that happen outside of therapy. Participants in group CBT for psychosis often have difficulties completing their homework, either because of the idea of homework, as mentioned previously, or because they simply forget the assignment or lack the motivation to complete it. From our experience, homework compliance changes according to the type of homework proposed—some participants shy away from paper-and-pencil homework but are quite willing to practice new behaviors as homework, whereas for others the opposite is true. To promote homework, therapists can reinforce those who have completed their homework at the beginning of each session by offering them a few minutes of individual attention while going over the assignment. It is also important to encourage those who have not done their homework by reviewing with them what would help them complete it (such as asking for someone in their household to remind them). In our group CBT for psychosis, the homework is given once every two sessions, allowing each participant sufficient time to complete it.

Therapy as a pleasurable experience: One of the essential therapeutic elements of group CBT for psychosis is that the group experience is a pleasurable one, even fun. This may sound odd to some therapists who were taught that therapy should trigger negative emotions that need to be worked through in therapy, or that therapy should focus on problems, not on having fun. Try to imagine having a diagnosis of schizophrenia, often having people telling you what to do or what they think is wrong with you, and being asked to take part in a group therapy with strangers that will also focus on trying to fix what is wrong with you. Who would want to attend if each session focused on distressing experiences and problems, with a serious therapist? These groups would likely increase feelings of uneasiness and distress and would definitely not entice people to return. Friendly groups, in which each session ends on a positive note, where even humor is evident during the sessions, and that help people connect and relate, are more likely to have higher participation and attendance. Group CBT for psychosis was developed to be delivered in such a manner. Although difficult experiences and themes are addressed, they are addressed carefully and ensure that people leave the group feeling OK, or better. At times, laughter and humor can occur, but they are never aimed at ridiculing someone. The mood of course has to be session-syntonic, meaning that it is appropriate to act light-hearted and more enthusiastic during a session that focuses on self-esteem but to be more neutral or serious during a session on suicidal thoughts. It is therefore understandable that group CBT for psychosis sessions focus not only on negative experiences (as mentioned previously) but also on positive qualities, goals, strengths, and protective factors. Also, the socialization period at the end of each session allows for friendly conversations to occur and for the group's experience to always end positively.

Conclusion

Although it has been years since Yalom's first descriptions and study of the essential elements of group psychotherapy, many of those elements remain central today. As this chapter has described, group psychotherapy is effective when these elements are taken into consideration and encouraged. Group cohesion and normalization, for instance, are particularly central when working with people with psychosis. Other elements, not mentioned by Yalom, are also relevant when delivering group CBT for psychosis, namely, offering a safe, structured, and positive group experience, as well as designing sessions that achieve small and specific goals, within a single-session time frame. Each of these elements contributes to the effectiveness of group CBT for psychosis, but they do not constitute the entire picture. Essential therapeutic elements are sine qua non elements in the sense that the therapy cannot be effective without them, yet they do not completely constitute what group CBT for psychosis is either. The following chapters will present in greater detail the specific techniques used in group CBT for psychosis, which, along with the essential elements presented here, can be considered the essence of group CBT for psychosis.

The Role of the Therapist in Group CBT for Psychosis

The therapist has a very different role in group therapy than in individual therapy. This chapter presents how to work in co-therapy, how to use the participants' input as ways to support the therapist, and what is expected of the therapist (e.g., show and ensure understanding, manage time and interactions, encourage group cohesion), as well as what he or she should watch out for and avoid (e.g., imposing his view, acting as an expert, monopolizing the session).

How Is the Therapist's Role Different in Group Than in Individual Therapy?

A therapist might be an expert in CBT for psychosis in individual therapy but might not be able to apply this knowledge to a group setting mainly because of the differences related to the role of the therapist and the lack of understanding of the group processes (mentioned in the previous chapter). For instance, in individual therapy, the therapist is entirely focused on the client, focusing on his or her goals and issues and suggesting ideas or techniques accordingly. In a group, a CBT for psychosis therapist will not focus in depth on each individual in turn (that would be like offering multiple small individual sessions in front of an audience) because it would be boring for the other participants and could feel intrusive for the person concerned. The therapist will instead offer themes and techniques that all participants could use and help each find a way to personalize them, while keeping the entire group interested and involved. Although each participant can share information or experiences and is encouraged to talk at various moments during the session, the therapist makes sure that each personal intervention is not too long and that everyone gets to participate. In this sense, the therapist acts somewhat like an

orchestra conductor: ensuring that everyone works together well and that each participant is getting the most out of every session.

In individual therapy, the therapist will also spend sufficient time on an issue for the
client to find his or her own answers at his or her own pace. In a group, we cannot adjust the
session's material to everybody's pace in the same way and at times might need to suggest
leads or answers for the group to move forward. When, as sometimes happens, everyone
in the group is unsure about their comprehension of a concept or how to answer a question, the group therapist will offer an answer as an example. In many ways the therapist
contributes in the group like the other participants, keeping in mind he or she not is only
facilitating normalization by sharing similar experiences (explained in Chapter 4) but also
is serving as a role model. This also means that the therapist uses reflective-self-disclosure.
It is reflective in the sense that it is thought through, has a purpose, and reveals some personal information but not enough for the participants to worry about the therapist's well-
being. For example, during the first sessions that focus on stress, the therapist might offer,
"I know I am stressed out when I feel my heart beating really fast and I can't think straight"
as a personal illustration to help others follow along and share their responses. At times, the
therapist's participation and self-disclosure might be used to help participants see things in
another way, especially positively. For example, when asked what could explain why a bus
driver is staring at you, instead of offering a paranoid response, the therapist might say, "The
bus driver is looking at me—probably he finds me attractive or well dressed." Or if participants speak of drinking or using drugs to cope with stress or symptoms, the therapist might
comment, "For me, I find I feel worse the next day if I drink too much. I often find it helps
me to call someone close and talk about what I'm going through instead."

In individual therapy, the therapist works at creating an alliance with the client, trying to engage him or her in the therapy by displaying warmth and understanding while
the client shares difficult personal information. In group therapy, the therapist also tries
to develop an alliance with each participant but works mostly on creating group cohesion
(described in Chapter 4). However, group cohesion is facilitated by not going too quickly
into difficult personal issues but instead working slowly on useful but not overly threatening topics before addressing more difficult topics. The therapist's role is therefore to ensure
the group exists as an entity first, before cognitive and behavior changes are introduced.

Finally, in individual therapy, if a personal problem arises or a relational problem
between the client and the therapist develops, it can be discussed immediately in the here
and now. In the group, the problem might need to be addressed both individually and
with the group, depending on its nature. For instance, if a conflict arises between two participants, the therapist might meet with each participant alone first before addressing the
issue with the entire group. This often means waiting until the end of the session, when
the other participants leave. Following the individual meeting and some form of resolution of the problem, and depending on the problem, perhaps a group apology will be
given without more details; at other times (especially when the group has a strong cohesion), more details about what happened might be shared with everyone in the group.

What Are the Differences Regarding the Role of the Therapist in Group CBT for Psychosis Compared With Other Group Approaches for People With Psychosis?

The main differences between the role of the therapist in group CBT for psychosis and in most other group approaches for people with psychosis can be summarized by two concepts: *expert* and *participant*. In most group approaches for people with psychosis, the therapist adopts an expert stance, clearly signifying to the group members that he or she is the holder of knowledge and is the expert in the room. This expert stance is recommended, for instance, for therapists using the Tavistock method (psychodynamic), who will intervene by stating or interpreting what they think is happening in the group at different moments (e.g., "You are all talking about your upcoming vacation. What are you really trying to avoid talking about?"; Semmelhack, Ende, & Hazell, 2013). In skills training, for instance (Liberman, 1992), this expertise is clearly conveyed by the therapist, who shows the participants how to perform a certain behavior and coaches them in imitating that behavior. In psychoeducation groups, the therapist may appear like a teacher in many ways and often leads the group like a classroom. In group CBT for psychosis, in contrast, the therapist is not the expert. Instead, this approach puts the therapist and the clients on the same level. The clients are experts on their experiences that they share with the group, whereas the therapist has some useful knowledge that he or she also shares. The therapist does not hold the "truth" or the "right way" to do things but brings another perspective and explains and shares it in a flexible way.

The second difference between group approaches in psychosis is the participant concept. In many psychodynamic groups, the therapist is more of an observer than an active participant. In such groups, the therapist intervenes only occasionally, to offer some interpretation of or reflection on what is going on, but otherwise is more passive and observant. In more behavioral groups, the therapists are the opposite, participating actively and intensively and guiding the group throughout each session. In group CBT for psychosis, the therapist is also an active participant but, given that he or she does not act as an expert, will make sure the participants are also active, helping each other and intervening frequently, during the sessions.

Co-therapy: An essential Part of Group CBT for Psychosis

There are divergent views regarding co-therapy, with some therapists suggesting it is not needed if the group is small but others stressing that it is essential. We tend to agree with the latter and strongly believe in the value of having two therapists conduct a group. One of the reasons is that not all individuals relate to everyone in the same way, and some might find it easier to communicate with one therapist more than with the other. Also, problems can arise in group therapy, even if the sessions are fairly structured as in group CBT for psychosis, and a co-therapist can ensure that the group continues on the task at hand while the other therapist deals with a problem (e.g., by leaving the group with one participant). We mentioned in the previous chapter that co-therapy with therapists of different gender is ideal, although it is not always possible. This is not only for modeling reasons but also because participants might have more difficulty relating to people from one gender or the other (because of past traumas or other experiences).

Co-therapy is an art! The choice of a co-therapist and how the co-therapists work together will strongly predict the success of the therapy. It is important for co-therapists to complement each other, being neither too similar nor too different in therapeutic style. This means, for instance, that a therapist who talks a lot and tends to lead the sessions will work best with someone who is more discreet, empathic, and able to encourage participants to talk. Two people with similar energy and therapeutic styles can also work well together, as long as they alternate their roles for each session. For instance, for one session, one therapist prepares the content, structures the session, and keeps track of time, while the other assists by engaging the participants and helping them understand and participate. The next session would be the opposite (the other therapist prepares and structures the session, etc.). This formula also helps balance out preparation time for each session, not overburdening a single therapist with the preparation for all the sessions. Co-therapists also need to take time not only before each session, to prepare and discuss the session's theme and how it will be carried out, but also at the end of each session, to debrief. We recommend that the co-therapists take notes together at the end of each session. A grid, which lists each participant's name and provides a space to code how they participated during the session (see the participation rating scale in the Appendix 4), allows co-therapists to recognize aspects of the interactions they might have missed during the session. This post-therapy rating time also provides an ideal opportunity to reflect on their own performance, that is, if they felt they did well or perhaps made mistakes or could have been more effective. Doing this immediately after the session will help in planning the next session, at times indicating a need to return to material that might have been explained too rapidly or awkwardly.

Essential Roles of the Therapist in Group CBT for Psychosis: The "To-Do" List

Box 5.1 summarizes some essential roles of the therapist in group CBT for psychosis, or what we call the "to-do" list.

BOX 5.1 To Do

1. Establish a good alliance and group cohesion.
2. Set treatment goals with person.
3. Offer a stable and consistent structure for the therapy.
4. Try to understand person's beliefs.
5. Work on the most distressing beliefs first.
6. Protect and enhance self-esteem.
7. Help person to discover his or her best ways of coping.
8. Promote the use of homework between sessions.

We have already mentioned the importance establishing a good alliance and good group cohesion. This is the first essential role of the therapist, given that without strong group cohesion and a good therapeutic alliance between each participant and the therapist, the participants will not benefit optimally from the content. As described in Chapter 4, the alliance and group cohesion will make the group a safe enough place to explore difficult topics and help participants agree to try changing their beliefs and behaviors. How does one establish a good alliance and good group cohesion? In addition to the elements we mentioned in Chapter 4, this question is also answered by taking time to get to know each participant before, during, and after each session. The alliance slowly builds as the therapists ask questions and show interest and caring. Also, by offering a treatment that makes sense to the participants, the therapists convey that the group answers a need. The alliance will develop naturally as the therapists demonstrate that this group intervention is useful, and that the therapists and participants will be "in the same boat," that is, working together, side by side. Group cohesion is facilitated by the choice of participants (described in detail in Chapter 6), by the use of activities that encourage positive interactions between participants, by the therapists making links between participants' responses and experiences, and by the socialization period at the end of each group.

The second role of the therapist is to set clear goals for the therapy and for each session. Although the session themes and goals can be predetermined (as is the case when using the workbook), it is still important to describe these goals, stress their importance, and verify if the participants agree that they are important goals to work on. Some sessions, for instance, on substance abuse, might not be considered relevant if no one in the group has or has had issues with drugs or alcohol. Therefore, that session could be modified to address other issues that are more central for the participants (e.g., dealing with compulsive or addictive behaviors such as overeating). If the goal of each session is clear and feasible, participants will have a sense of accomplishment at the end of the session because they have met that goal.

The third important role of the therapist is to offer a stable and consistent structure for the group sessions. This essentially means that the sessions are similar enough that participants have an idea of what to expect. The group always starts at the same time, ends at the same time, happens on the same days, is run by the same co-therapists, and follows a similar structure. Each session starts with a recapitulation of what has been accomplished so far, followed by a review of the last session, a description of the current session (goal), and the session itself (activity—questions, discussions); it finishes with a review of the goal, a discussion of what each participant wishes to remember, and the socialization period. This stable structure makes the group feel safe, which, as described in Chapter 4, is one of the essential ingredients for therapeutic effectiveness.

The fourth role of the therapist is to try to understand the participants' beliefs. This may sound easy, but some individuals with psychosis might have difficulties expressing their beliefs, which in turn can make it even harder for the therapist to grasp the meaning and implications of the beliefs. For instance, one participant incessantly repeated that he had not killed his mother. Was this a belief or a fact? (The therapy was taking place in a forensic unit/ward, so it was possible that he had actually killed her.) Did he kill his mother and now was feeling guilty? Was his mother fine, but he was frightened by his own violence? Did he witness someone hurting his mother? Or, in another example, a participant mentioned her food being poisoned. What did this mean? Did she find the food had an odd taste? (Perhaps her medication changed her sense of taste.) Did she think people were out to get her and wished her dead (because of something she did, or because she had special powers and they were jealous)? To try to understand the participant's belief, the therapist takes the time to ask, "What does it say about you?" or "Why is that happening to you?" and does not simply accept the belief or statement at face value. This understanding will of course influence the strategies that will be used to help the person change the belief or feel less distressed about it. For instance, the participant who believed her food was being poisoned because the food tasted strange was really distressed because she could not understand why this was happening to her—she had never harmed anyone and did not feel she was special in any way. She was, however, open to seeking alternative explanations (such as that her medication was affecting her taste buds) more readily than if the belief had been linked to prosecution or grandiosity.

This leads us to the next role: Always work on the most distressing beliefs first. Therapists, especially those who know the participants well from seeing them during their hospitalization or following them as case managers, often have their own agenda for what the participants should work on during the group. For instance, one participant was considered quite annoying by many mental health members because he believed he was extremely rich and that the hospital was withholding his money from him. This was considered to be a delusion, and the therapist in training was hoping to use the group CBT for psychosis to modify this belief. However, that was not the participant's goal in the therapy—he was not distressed by his belief of being rich. He was more preoccupied by not having friends and not being liked by others. Often clinicians wrongly think that CBT for psychosis should focus exclusively on psychotic symptoms. It actually targets distressing symptoms and dysfunctional beliefs, which are not necessarily always related to psychotic symptoms. Of course, the participant who believes he is very rich is alienating himself by bragging about his wealth and harassing the mental health staff for his money; his behavior is contributing to his difficulty in making friends and feeling liked. However, it is best to present the goal of making friends first and then see how he can change his behavior to help reach that goal. In the end, the behaviors related to his belief about being rich will change, although the belief will not have been addressed from the start. We do not address the belief up front because (a) it does not cause him obvious distress, and (b) it appears to be linked to his self-esteem (I am rich = I have self-worth).

The next important role of the therapist is therefore to protect and enhance the participants' self-esteem. The group CBT for psychosis module we use includes self-esteem activities that aim at helping participants recognize their positive qualities and modify their negative attributional styles. Feelings of being an important group member and meeting goals in the group also help enhance a participant's self-esteem. It is important to be aware of interventions that might be harmful for the person's self-esteem; for example, it is best not to propose CBT techniques that attempt to directly modify grandiose beliefs. At times, the belief clearly appears linked to self-esteem: The participant mentions having special powers and appears proud of them. It is not indicated to "seek facts" or try to change that belief directly because those powers appear to make the participant feel special and are likely linked to his or her self-esteem. At other times, however, the grandiosity is not as obvious. Someone might describe being followed by secret agents from the government; that belief might bring distress ("They might wish to hurt me") or might be grandiose ("I am so important that they want me"). The former could be addressed more readily than the latter. We do not want to remove the belief that anyone in the group is special in any way; we do, however, wish to help participants discover how they can truly be special, without needing the grandiose belief to feel good about themselves.

The therapist should also help each participant discover his or her own best ways of coping. There is no single good way to cope with stress or specific symptoms. What works for one therapist or for one participant might not work for another. People with psychosis often already use a number of coping strategies—some effectively and some less so. The goal is to help enlarge that repertoire so they have more than one option they know will work for them. There is no use in pushing participants to exercise or take part in sports when they are feeling overstressed if they do not enjoy exercise. We have a list of coping strategies that we offer, with room for extra suggestions from the group, to encourage participants to try new strategies. The therapist's role is to help participants try different coping strategies and figure out which ones work best for them, and in which context (e.g., "It might help to call my mom if I'm not feeling well, but not while I'm at work").

Finally, the therapist must find ways to encourage participants to do their homework. Homework enables participants to integrate what was done during the group in their real-life context. As mentioned in Chapter 4, most homework suggested in the group CBT for psychosis workbook essentially repeats concepts or techniques introduced in the session, but the participants are asked to use examples from their week.

Mistakes to Avoid: The Do-Not List

The CBT for psychosis therapist should avoid acting in certain ways and adopting specific attitudes that are described in the following box. The 'Do-Not' list is not exhaustive. It does however illustrate mistakes that we have witnessed during our workshops or supervision sessions.

BOX 5.2 The "Do-Not" List

1. Act as an expert.
2. Impose your view or your formulation of the patient's issues.
3. Try to convince the person to see things differently.
4. Aim at modifying the psychotic symptoms at all costs.
5. Demean a person's belief as "only a symptom of your illness" or show stigmatizing attitudes.
6. Be inconsistent or interpretative.
7. Apply CBT techniques at random.
8. Monopolize the group discussion.
9. Use CBT for psychosis without appropriate training and supervision.

Essentially, all the items in the "to-do" list, if presented as the opposite, can become "do-not" elements, and thus they do not need to be repeated here. But the first mistake to avoid is acting like an expert. In fact, the opposite—maintaining a modest demeanor—is preferred. We recommend that first-time group CBT for psychosis therapists tell their participants that it is their first time running this group. Therapists should mention how they will be working together, and that the group will be a shared learning experience. Acting as an expert will create an imbalance in the group, a "me" and "them" instead of "us."

The second mistake the therapist should avoid is imposing his or her view or formulation of the participants' issues. The therapist might have an idea of the elements that have led to a specific participant's belief and the elements that sustain that belief, but if the participant does not agree and does not see the issues in the same way, there is no need to insist. The goal is to reach an understanding and an agreed-upon conceptualization of the participant's goals and issues. The therapist's formulation or views might be "right," but the participant might not be open to seeing things in that way. Or the therapist might be missing some information that might help explain why the participant disagrees with the therapist's view. Either way, it is best to find a compromise and work on a common understanding than to insist and risk breaking the alliance.

The next mistake follows along the same lines: Do not try to convince the participant to see things differently. Of course, group CBT for psychosis is meant to help people change their dysfunctional beliefs, but not by force. Some people might quickly be ready to change their beliefs and behaviors, whereas others might find it too threatening and will not be ready to see things differently. They might still benefit from the group CBT for psychosis, perhaps by trying to learn more coping strategies or becoming more trusting of others, but they might not be ready to work on changing their beliefs just yet. It is important to accept that not all participants will change their beliefs; some will not budge at all, others might only start doubting their beliefs, and some will undergo a complete transformation and will develop a different outlook on their beliefs during the group.

The fourth potential mistake is linked to trying to improve psychotic symptoms at all costs. As mentioned previously, some participants might present with psychotic symptoms but will wish to focus on other difficulties, whereas others will not be open to changing specific symptom-related beliefs.

The fifth mistake to avoid is using psychiatric labels to discredit the person's experience. Regardless of whether the discourse describes paranoid thoughts or a real situation, the person with the belief can experience true distress and fear. It is important to realize that using labels such as *delusion* or *hallucination* or saying that a belief is not real but is just a symptom of schizophrenia does not change the person's experience in a positive way. Most often, people will feel misunderstood and not believed. It is better to recognize the person's distress and to validate his or her experience, by saying, for example, "If I thought people were out to kill me, I would also be very scared." With such a comment, we are not stating in any way that the experience is "real" or "unreal," but we are still validating the participant's experience.

The sixth mistake to avoid is being inconsistent or interpretative. Although most participants can accept it if their therapists undergo some minor changes during the group, consistency is best. We typically recommend that changing one's hair color or shaving a beard should be done prior to starting the group, not in the middle of it. Similarly, therapists are expected to be "real" and authentic, which also means being fairly stable and consistent in their attitudes from one session to the next. As for avoiding interpretations, group CBT for psychosis does not aim at uncovering the exact historical reason for a particular delusion in each participant but instead focuses on change, solutions, and coping strategies. Of course, to formulate or personalize an understanding of their distressing thoughts, some explanations will arise, but the focus of the session should not linger on these. Most cognitive behavioral therapists will agree that understanding the origin of one's problems is helpful, but concrete behavioral and cognitive changes make a bigger difference in the person's life.

The seventh mistake to avoid is using CBT for psychosis techniques at random. Many clinicians, when they start looking at the sessions and activities in the workbook (provided in the Appendix 1) will want to use only some sessions with their clients, perhaps even in individual therapy. Clinicians might be attracted to activities that come up later in the workbook and could even wish to use them first or alone. For some activities, this might be OK (such as self-esteem activities), but most sessions were designed to be offered in a specific order, and the techniques are therefore introduced in a logical manner. To use any random session or technique might simply not be effective if the necessary groundwork has not been covered. Furthermore, the workbook has been validated "as is," with its 24 sessions, and we do not know how effective the individual sessions are by themselves. Another issue regarding the order of CBT techniques has to do with the acceptability of the technique by participants. We know, for instance, that having a new model for understanding one's issues (either via formulation or by personalizing the stress-vulnerability-competence model) and having experienced normalization in the group are necessary prior to attempting any belief modification. Changing beliefs and behaviors can be very challenging for many individuals with psychosis, and this needs to be addressed tactfully and at the right moment.

The eighth mistake is for therapists to monopolize the group discussions. Some therapists might have previous experience in running psychoeducation or skills training groups and could therefore be inclined to act like teachers. Some groups might also include participants who are less verbal or who have more negative symptoms, which may also create in some therapists the need to "fill the void" and do most of the talking. Although we do not recommend long silences, the therapist's role is to find various ways to get the participants in the group to talk, ensuring that everyone participates. In Chapter 12, we will present strategies that can help in working with less verbal clients.

Finally, it is important that only therapists who have received the appropriate training conduct group CBT for psychosis. In Chapter 13, we discuss the specific skills that are needed, but essentially, to offer group CBT for psychosis, it is best that the therapists either have received specific group CBT for psychosis training or have experience in conducting group therapy with people with psychosis and have a strong understanding of the CBT principles and techniques. A therapist with previous training in individual CBT for psychosis might also be able to conduct group CBT for psychosis but would most likely need a co-therapist who has group experience. We have found that clinicians who have experience in delivering individual CBT for psychosis tend to have more difficulties in learning to conduct a group than group therapists without prior CBT for psychosis experience have in learning to deliver group CBT for psychosis. However, motivated therapists who are willing to change their framework and to acquire new skills can successfully conduct group CBT for psychosis, especially when following the workbook (provided in the Appendix 1).

Conclusion

This chapter has explained the unique role of therapists in group CBT for psychosis. The guidelines offered here might initially seem complex and numerous, especially when one is working with many individuals together in a group context, but they will quickly become natural as clinicians gather experience in group CBT for psychosis. It might be difficult for participants to accept that their therapists are not "experts" who will prescribe the best strategies for feeling better. Yet the shared learning will empower participants to have greater faith in their own capacity to overcome their difficulties and meet their goals. The therapists' role essentially encompasses the necessary therapeutic attitudes to apply CBT for psychosis techniques. The following chapters will describe these techniques chronologically, as presented in the workbook.

6

Getting Started

This chapter covers all that needs to be put in place prior to starting the group and how to ensure attendance. We have mentioned the importance of co-therapy in a previous chapter. Here, we will discuss what needs to be considered in terms of recruitment, selection of participants, the choice of the setting, the schedule and frequency of sessions, use of a participant manual, materials and snacks, and dealing with transportation issues, missed sessions, measuring outcomes, and so forth.

Recruitment

Although group CBT for psychosis is typically greatly appreciated by participants, recruiting people to take part in a new group can be a challenge. Psychosis is associated with negative symptoms such as lack of motivation, which can be challenging for ensuring attendance at any therapy, and whereas people with anxiety might line up to receive a treatment, and may even be willing to have their names on a waiting list for months, recruiting people with psychosis for therapy can be much more difficult. Various strategies might need to be considered according to the setting.

In inpatient settings (or group homes/supervised apartments) where most participants reside in the same setting, recruitment can be facilitated by meeting each participant a few weeks before the first group session to explain the purpose of the group and discuss how it might help participants meet their personal goals. Large posters indicating the dates of the group, frequent reminders of the start of the group, and having the group therapist seek out each participant a few minutes before the first session are useful strategies. Inpatient or residential settings have the advantage of access to participants; consequently, it can be easier to recruit enough participants to start a group. One disadvantage is that the participants know each other, which might affect group cohesion if some refuse to take part if a specific participant is present. Recruiting in such a context is facilitated by prior knowledge of the setting's dynamics and issues. Of course, the group might help resolve a conflict between two participants, but it is best to be aware of the conflict and perhaps prepare the participants during the recruitment phase so they know who they will meet during the group.

In outpatient settings within the public system, recruitment implies the collaboration of the entire clinical team. Given that potential participants might come to the clinic only for occasional appointments, each clinician needs to mention the group to his or her clients, perhaps handing out flyers that describe the group and how they might benefit from it. It is the group therapist's job to remind the other clinicians often about the upcoming group and encourage their participation in the recruitment phase. Posters in the waiting area can also attract people's attention. The clinician or group therapist also needs to follow up on potential participants' interest by phone and ideally meet them in person prior to the first group meeting to ensure the group is a good fit for them. Recruiting future group participants in the community might take some time; as a consequence, some individuals might change their mind and no longer wish to participate when the group is ready to start. It is therefore preferable to recruit more participants to begin with (e.g., 10 or 12), even if the goal is to run a group of 6 to 8 participants.

Recruiting participants for group CBT for psychosis within a research context is actually quite similar to recruiting for inpatients or outpatients, with the difference that the research team is rarely fully integrated with the clinical team. As a consequence, it might be more difficult to obtain clinicians' collaboration during the recruitment phase. One possible solution is to include one of the setting's clinicians as a co-therapist, thereby ensuring closer collaboration with the clinicians as well as greater knowledge transfer once the study is completed. Clinicians are more likely to agree to participate in a study if they feel there is an "added value" for them or their clients. Offering free training sessions on how to conduct group CBT for psychosis has been an incentive for clinicians to participate and help with the recruitment in our studies. For potential participants, a small stipend for their time spent completing questionnaires and tests before and after the group is also a good incentive.

Recruiting participants for group CBT for psychosis in a private setting requires different strategies. At times, public settings might not offer individual or group CBT for psychosis, and parents of individuals with psychosis, or the individuals themselves, might seek psychological help privately. It is rare, however, that a large enough number of potential participants to conduct a group will seek private help at the same time. A private psychotherapist who wishes to conduct group CBT for psychosis would therefore need to develop links with the area's public clinics in order to publicize the upcoming group and obtain referrals. Community organizations, particularly mental health organizations and parent support organizations, should also be contacted to develop ties and to send them publicity for the group. Potential participants need to be met individually before deciding if the group format would be appropriate or not for each person, according to his or her needs. For the participants seeking private therapy, the group format has the advantage of costing significantly less per session than individual private therapy.

Selection of Participants

One of the most frequently encountered questions during group CBT for psychosis workshops is "How do you select participants?" This question implies several underlying questions, such as "Who will benefit most?, "Who will work well together?," and "Who might not be able to tolerate a group?" In the context of our past studies on group CBT for psychosis, typically we would recommend that clinicians not select participants but simply refer anyone who fits our inclusion criteria (i.e., presented with psychotic symptoms) and who wishes to participate. As described in Chapter 3, some preliminary studies suggest that participants with certain traits or profiles might gain more than others from CBT for psychosis or group CBT for psychosis. Yet these studies have not consistently found the same results, suggesting that there are no clear indications of who will benefit or not. For instance, a participant in one of our groups had several catatonic symptoms when he started the group, barely spoke or moved, and was not taking his prescribed psychiatric medication. After a few sessions, in which he heard from others how medication was a protective factor for them, he started following his prescription and soon became more alert and sociable; eventually, after the group ended, he was able to continue working toward completing his college degree. It is important to remember that the group can have therapeutic effects even if the person has not entirely grasped all the CBT for psychosis concepts and techniques. The essential group elements presented in Chapter 4 can lead many to have a positive group experience even if only a few of the techniques or concepts are applied in their daily lives. Furthermore, some participants will retain only a single concept (e.g., the vulnerability-stress-competence model) or a single coping strategy (e.g., the relaxation technique), but they will describe this new knowledge as having had a positive impact on their lives. The selection of participants should therefore not be based on a priori notions regarding who might benefit from the therapy. It should be based on a second question: "Who will work well together?"

This second question refers to the concepts of homogeneity or heterogeneity among the group's participants. Homogeneous groups are typically preferred, although not necessarily in terms of clinical presentation so much as in terms of functioning. Similarly, some participants might hear voices, whereas others might present with more persecutory or grandiose thoughts, but they still might be able to develop strong group cohesion. However, functioning will affect the pace and cohesion of the group. Functioning can imply social functioning, such as the ability to talk and be an active participant in the group, but here we mostly mean cognitive functioning. When part of the group is highly educated and quickly grasps concepts, and the other members have important cognitive deficits and struggle to understand, ensuring that everyone gets the most out of the group becomes extremely challenging for the therapists. It is therefore recommended, when possible, to try to bring together people with similar cognitive functioning. Although cognitive assessments are not always available in clinical settings, education levels can be a good indication of cognitive functioning.

Age is another important factor to consider. It can be difficult to conduct a group with participants from different age groups, particularly if a minority of participants are at one extreme and the rest of the participants are at the other extreme of the age range. An 18-year-old participant who has recently experienced a first psychotic episode and is struggling with substance abuse and peer pressure might not feel comfortable taking part in a group with people over 40 with longer mental illness experience. Similarly, an older participant might feel "old" and set apart if most group members are much younger. Older people with years of institutionalization can scare younger individuals, leading them to lose hope, doubt the possibility of their own recovery, and fear that they too might end up with severe deficits and never lead a fulfilling life. Ideally, participants should be more or less within 10 years of age of each other; this is especially the case when working with youth or young adults. However, this criterion becomes less important among older individuals (e.g., late 30s and older), who tend to have a greater ability to relate to people of different ages.

Last but not least, personality problems need to be considered when selecting participants for a group. People with psychosis can also present with personality disorders, and some participants might be more disruptive than others. Although it is possible to run a group with some participants who present with borderline, narcissistic, or antisocial traits as well as psychosis, it is important to keep in mind that such a group might be challenging for a novice therapist. It is therefore important for therapists to be aware of participants' personality profiles to decide if they feel sufficiently skilled to include these individuals in the group. Meeting each participant prior to beginning the group might help in making this decision. We will address how to work with more difficult participants in Chapter 12.

Finally, the third question regarding the person's ability to tolerate a group can be easily answered. Participants who feel they cannot benefit from or attend group therapy will simply not show up or will abandon the group after the first or second session. As mentioned previously, the groups should be voluntary. Someone who feels overstressed in a group situation, because of social anxiety, paranoia, or other issues, is always free to refuse to attend or discontinue the group. Typically, 2 out of 10 participants will leave the group after the first or second session. To our knowledge, to date no one has ever experienced negative effects from attending group CBT for psychosis.

Choosing the Setting and Schedule

Choosing the setting and schedule might not be an issue for groups conducted in a residential or inpatient setting, given that clinicians have access to everyone's weekly schedule and are therefore able to propose a time and location during free periods when most participants are available.

For people living in the community, finding the right schedule and setting can be more difficult. The group should be conducted when everyone is available, which might mean in the evening. Many clinicians or clinical settings do not provide services after 5:00 p.m., yet offering the group during the day might mean losing potential participants who work or attend school. Clinicians might be available in the morning, for instance, but some participants might be unable to attend if they struggle to leave their beds because of medication side effects. Furthermore, some potential participants might be attending school or working during the day. Therapists wishing to offer groups should take these factors into consideration and might need to negotiate their own work schedules to maximize participant recruitment and attendance, such as by finishing later one or two days a week. In terms of setting, a fixed group room that remains available for the entire length of the group is ideal. The room should be spacious enough to seat up to 12 people but small enough to feel cozy. It is important for the room to be comfortable, with windows and enough space for people to not feel trapped or confined. Ideally, the room should include a table, around which participants sit, enabling them to comfortably write in their workbooks.

Frequency and Length of Sessions

Most of our groups with participants living in the community run twice a week for 3 months, for a total of 24 hourly sessions. This session frequency has many advantages. If someone misses a session, the next one will not be too far away, making it easier to catch up with the rest of the group. It is also less difficult to remember the content of a session that happened only a few days earlier. Most participants can maintain their attention for 50 minutes, making the 60-minute session a good length. Psychologically, and especially for youth and young adults, a 3-month program resembles a semester at school and is therefore not perceived as a great time commitment. If possible, this is the recommended format.

For some participants and clinicians, however, a single session per week might be perceived as preferable. Some participants might have to travel long distances to attend the group sessions and might prefer sessions that are longer in duration but less frequent. Clinicians working as co-therapists might not be available more than once a week to deliver a group together. Some settings prefer to offer two 1-hour sessions, with a break in the middle, but only once a week. Others have chosen to offer only a single session per week (stretching it to last up to 90 minutes) but over the course of 6 months. The 2-hour groups have been successful with people with higher levels of cognitive functioning, whereas 6-month/once-a-week groups have been more popular with participants who were somewhat older, a bit slower in learning, and not deterred by longer treatments.

We have also used a briefer, 16-session version of our group CBT for psychosis manual for people who were temporarily hospitalized. This format involves three to four sessions per week over the course of 4 to 6 weeks. When using this format, it is important to include a smaller number of participants (maximum four) given that their symptoms might be overwhelming for some, and each participant might need more assistance during the sessions. The sessions used for this format are detailed in the manual (see Appendix 3).

Manual or Workbook

The importance of using a manual or workbook, which enables participants to prepare for themes that will be covered in future sessions, has been mentioned previously. The value of offering a manual at the first session cannot be emphasized enough. Some clinicians are used to giving handouts, but these will not have the same impact, since they are most often given at each session and not in advance. The manual is also a tool, allowing participants to read and review concepts, as well as giving them space to write down their thoughts and answers. Participants might not wish to share everything they have written, but they will be able to reflect on their experience and refer to the manual when needed. The manual also helps people with memory difficulties to remember what they have worked on during past sessions. Therapists should be sufficiently prepared prior to each session to conduct the group using the same manual or workbook as the participants, without needing the support of the clinician's supplement (or of this book). It is possible that participants will forget their workbook at home; in such cases, spare copies of the session in the workbook can be used and brought home. Some participants who fear forgetting their workbook at home between sessions might ask to leave it with the therapists and only tear out the homework pages to take home.

Materials and Snacks

Having some materials available for use at sessions can facilitate group CBT for psychosis. A flip chart can be used at almost every session to write some of the participants' answers or to illustrate techniques, models, or principles. A blackboard or whiteboard can also be used, but the flip chart allows the group to revisit elements that have been mentioned previously, when needed (such as group rules or models). One session asks for each participant to write his or her answers on a flip chart page; it is important to have enough markers for everyone during that session.

A box of pencils should also be made available for participants to write in their workbooks. Some items are needed for a single session, such as video clips showing examples of wrong conclusions being drawn based on partial information (various examples can be found online, or movie excerpts can also be used—we give suggestions in Chapter 8). These can be shown on a television or computer screen. Yoga mats, gym mats, or cushions can also be used for the session on relaxation. We strongly recommend having a small snack available at the end of the session, ideally juice, tea, or coffee to drink and something fairly nutritious to eat (fruits, nuts, granola bars). Some settings might not have a budget for snacks, but we recommend providing them, if possible, because they encourage people to stay and socialize for 10 to 15 minutes after the group.

Transportation

Groups conducted with community participants may face transport issues. If participants live in a large urban area, most of them will have access to public transportation. Having enough resources to pay for transportation may be a challenge for some, however; if the clinic is able to offer bus or metro passes, this obstacle can be easily overcome. Some participants will need to travel long distances to attend the group; for them, carpooling or meeting up to take public transportation together may be suggested to help improve attendance. Some participants, especially young adults, might be living with their parents, who might be willing to drive the participant to his or her group. Some years ago it was possible for group therapists to use their own car or a minivan to pick up participants before a group, ensuring that transportation would not be an obstacle. Such practices are rarely seen now, mostly for insurance reasons. An assessment of transportation issues and potential solutions needs to be considered prior to beginning the sessions.

Attendance

Besides transportation, other reasons for poor attendance are poor motivation and cognitive difficulties. The therapists can help with both issues by giving participants a reminder telephone call the day before the group and also boosting motivation by mentioning that they are looking forward to seeing them the next day. These friendly reminders can take place during the first 2 weeks, or even longer for those who might have more memory difficulties. When someone misses a session, one of the therapists should call the participant the same day to obtain a reason for the absence and to encourage the participant to attend the next one and to try to complete the session in the workbook by him- or herself. This is extremely important because, at times, participants might miss a session because of unfounded beliefs, and the therapists can help verify the facts and consider alternatives. For instance, a participant who believed that no one liked her was surprised and happy to hear from the therapist that everyone had inquired about her when she had missed a session.

We also recommend that the participant who has missed a session arrive a bit earlier for the following one so the therapists can take a few minutes to go over the essential elements covered during the missed session. By proceeding in this manner, the participant does not feel lost or left out and can easily reintegrate into the group. However, if a participant misses several sessions (e.g., more than six sessions in a row), regardless of the reason, we recommend that he or she begin with a new group rather than rejoin the original group but feel lost or left behind. In such cases, the group members should be informed of the reason for the missed sessions (e.g., hospitalization, physical illness, or a change in residence).

Avoiding Vacation Breaks

Time-limited groups, such as the group CBT for psychosis described here, yield the best results when they are offered intensively, that is, without missed sessions because of holidays or therapists taking vacations. Of course, it can be difficult to conduct a group without any interruptions, given that major holidays might occur over the course of 3 or 6 months. It is, however, best to begin a new group after a long holiday, either in September or in January or February, ensuring that the group will be completed before the next long holiday.

Measuring Outcomes

Many clinical settings do not automatically measure outcomes when they plan a group. Chapter 11 proposes various measures that can be administered quickly and that allow therapists and clinics to collate data to support running group CBT for psychosis. It is important to think ahead about which measures will be administered, at what time, and by whom, and to decide how the data will be collected and analyzed. There is no point in administering assessments if no one can enter or analyze the data and the assessments are left in boxes for years. However, short and targeted assessments are possible and recommended and require only limited resources (see Chapter 11).

Conclusion

This chapter has covered everything that therapists will need to consider before starting their group. Factors related to recruiting participants, planning the schedule, space, and materials, and anticipating potential obstacles to running the group were explored. The next chapters will cover how to run the group and the content of the sessions.

7

Stress: How It Affects Me (Sessions 1 to 6)

This chapter describes the initial six sessions of our workbook (found in the Appendix 1), which include setting the rules, the icebreaker activity, and introducing nonthreatening topics that are considered useful and make sense to participants. We also describe how the activities have been designed to engage people, help them relate to each other, and offer a new way of understanding their symptoms within the vulnerability-stress-competence model.

S-1 (Session 1): Introducing Ourselves

The first session is crucial because it will determine if participants will wish to engage in the treatment. As described in earlier chapters, participants will engage if they feel the treatment makes sense to them and answers a need but also if they feel they can relate to and trust the people in the group. The purpose of the first session is therefore twofold: to offer an overview of the content of group CBT for psychosis by stating the objectives of the group and explaining how the workbook is divided, and to help participants get to know each other. Once everyone has arrived, it is important for the therapists to introduce themselves and ask everyone to say their name. Then the therapists should explain that group CBT for psychosis aims to help participants develop new strategies to cope with their mental health. They should also indicate that each participant will receive his or her own workbook and mention the time and frequency of the group meetings. Before beginning the first workbook activity, everyone needs to agree on the group's rules.

The Rules

Setting the rules as a group ensures from the start that everyone agrees on how the group should be run. The basic rules in group CBT for psychosis are as follows:

- Everyone respects each other.
- No comment is ever judged as good or bad.
- Each participant has the right to speak (but might be interrupted if he or she is moving away from the topic being discussed or to let someone else speak).
- We avoid talking about others in the group when outside of the group (confidentiality). However, there are limits to confidentiality—for instance, if someone in the group is presenting behaviors or thoughts that are particularly worrying (such as suicidal thoughts), the appropriate people (e.g., clinical team) will be contacted.
- There is a time after the group for off-topic discussions (socialization/snack period).

Other rules that are often brought up by participants might include turning off mobile phones, being on time, not taking illicit drugs or alcohol before attending the group, and so forth. One rule that we recommend to add is that the group should be fun! Participants are often surprised by this rule, but the therapists can explain that they are here to work together, and even though at times topics might be difficult to discuss, they will try to make the experience as enjoyable as possible.

How to Use the Workbook

Some clinicians might not be used to conducting a group with a workbook and might fear that the therapy will resemble a classroom. The workbook can in fact be a useful tool, as participants can read the question and then be given enough time to think about and find their own answers before hearing what others have to say. The workbook proposed (reproduced in the Appendix 1) has a specific format: Each activity has a number (preceded by a letter corresponding to the title of the section, e.g., an "S" for the section on stress, a "T" for the section on testing hypotheses), a title, a brief summary or goal of the session, a number of questions (at times with text or with role plays or other learning tools), and finally a question regarding what each participant wishes to remember about the session. Typically, the best way to use the workbook would be as follows:

- Ask for a volunteer to read the top box that describes the activity (or ask someone by name if no one volunteers), then add details, repeat in your own words, or comment as needed. For example:

   T-4 HOW NOT-TO-JUMP TO CONCLUSIONS

   We often make interpretations or decisions based on very little facts. Yet, we have learned so far how it is easy to misinterpret an event or situation. Today, we will explore how to prove or disprove our hypotheses before jumping to conclusions.

- Ask for a volunteer to read other text and/or the first question and give everyone enough time to write down their answers.
- Go around the group and ask each person (asking for volunteers first) to share their answer, one at a time, and comment with "Very good," "Yes, that is often true," or "Did

anyone else write something similar?," or gently use questioning to redirect the answer if pertinent.

- Ask a different person to read each question. If a question was answered in the previous discussion, it can be skipped.
- At the end of the session, review what was said, make a link with the theme of the activity, and ask clients to write down what they wish to remember (they can also share their answer with the group).
- Describe the homework (if applicable), then close the workbook and take some time to socialize and have a snack (if available).

Icebreaker

The first activity in the workbook is meant for people to get to know each other in a positive way. Participants (and therapists) are asked about where they live (not specifically but, for instance, the east or west part of the city or in a suburb), their favorite musician or band, their interests, a positive personal quality, and something they are good at. The session intentionally has a positive focus and does not address mental illness at all. Participants learn about each other as people with potential, qualities, and interests first. The discussion brings people to realize common interests and leads them to share their enthusiasm on topics of interest. Because the session started with an overview of the content of the group CBT for psychosis, as well as the group rules, the participants do not leave feeling they just talked about a general topic such as music. Most will leave feeling that the group might help them and that they might be able to connect with some of the other participants.

S-2 (Session 2): What Is Stress?

The second session aims to help participants understand what stress is and how it can have an impact on our emotions, thoughts, and bodies. At first glance, the session appears to start with a lot of theory, explaining the fight-or-flight reaction that is a response when facing danger and who initially studied and defined stress. By presenting this theoretical material, we convey the message that we believe the participants are smart enough to understand these concepts. It also allows the group members to participate without having to self-disclose too much. Given that it is only the second session, asking them to read and comment on a written text is not threatening and encourages participation. Furthermore, stress is a nonstigmatizing and fairly popular topic that affects everyone and can have a particularly important impact on one's mental health. It is the first building block in understanding the stress-vulnerability-competence model (see Chapter 2) that will be explained to participants in session 5.

To address how stress can be experienced, participants are first instructed, "Name an important event for you." The answer should portray a situation or context that the participant considers stressful. If it does not, the therapists should try to help the participant find another example of an important event that triggers stress. We then ask participants to keep their example in mind while answering the following questions on how stress can be experienced physically, in their mind, and by different emotions. This may seem obvious, but many of the symptoms listed can be experienced by participants as side effects of medication, for instance, and not necessarily be associated with stress. The list of potential symptoms can be read out loud, with both participants and therapists simply checking the items and raising a hand if they experience that specific symptom linked to stress. The goal is to help participants become more aware of when they are experiencing symptoms of stress. The activity also facilitates normalization by helping people realize that such symptoms are fairly common and are experienced by several participants in the group. In fact, the therapists themselves might experience very similar symptoms of stress, further adding to the normalization effect. The homework proposed is essentially to rate again symptoms of stress at home while thinking about another important stressful event.

S-3 (Session 3): What Do I Consider Stressful?

Once participants are able to recognize symptoms of stress, the next step is to recognize the situations, people, or contexts that might initiate a stressful response and help them self-rate their stress level. Session 3 helps participants identify situations, people, actions, or contexts that are repetitive or sporadic and that create symptoms of stress. This task may be difficult. Participants might feel extremely stressed when discussing money with their parents but will not recall that situation during the session. The therapists will sometimes need to give various examples to help participants find five different answers that apply to them (we do not wish for participants to identify only one example here). This task might take a bit of time to complete; it is suggested that the co-therapists each take some time with half of the participants, helping them individually with their answers, before having participants share their answers with the group. After discussing their answers (with feedback from the therapists, who at times point out similarities between different participants' answers), the participants are asked to choose one of their five answers and rate it as 0 to 7, according to the My Stress Level scale (Figure 7.1).

Each anchor point of the scale is carefully read and explained before asking participants to self-rate. This can be done with the entire group together, with a flip chart, using each participant's example and helping that person rate his or her stress level. The therapists point out that the anchor points on the scale are examples but that participants should also consider the symptoms of stress described during the previous session, asking them to recognize the symptoms that might indicate higher levels of stress for them. The homework is to complete the My Stress Level scale at home, using a stressful event the person experiences between sessions.

Level 0	**Feeling good** I am calm, at peace with myself.
Level 1	**Minimal stress** I feel a little nervous, or agitated. It is temporary and I don't mind.
Level 2	**Light stress** I feel a little discomfort and I am trying to understand what is going on.
Level 3	**Moderate stress** Effects on my body, mind and emotions, but I am still in control. I can go on.
Level 4	**Important stress** I feel strange, uncomfortable. My heart is pounding and my muscles are tense. I am trying to find out how to stay in control.
Level 5	**Anxiety** I don't breath easily, I'm feeling strange, or dizzy. I am afraid I am going to lose control. I want to run away.
Level 6	**Moderate anxiety** My heart is pounding, I feel disoriented, like if it was not real. I can't breath normally. I can't control myself any longer.
Level 7	**Panic** It is physically painful. I am afraid, I think I'm going to lose my mind. I am afraid of dying, I want to run away and escape right now.

FIGURE 7.1 My Stress Level scale.

S-4 (Session 4): How I Experience My Symptoms

When we initially tested out this module, we moved this session a few times before deciding on this place in the workbook. Participants had mentioned they were eager to find out if other participants had experienced similar symptoms to theirs but did not feel comfortable discussing symptoms earlier in the program. Session 4 is the preferred timing for allowing people to share their experience of hospitalization or of psychiatric symptoms.

This session has multiple goals. The first and most obvious is to enable people to share and connect with others, realizing they have experienced similar symptoms or feelings. This sharing not only is normalizing but also helps strengthen the group's cohesion. Even though the answers often describe negative events or distress, participants are happy to learn that others have had similar experiences. The therapists do not intervene using CBT techniques here—we do not emphasize normalization or try to explore alternatives or induce doubt. The session is about sharing common experiences between participants, and for therapists to gain an understanding of how the participants make sense of their experiences.

The second goal is to set the groundwork for an alternative explanation (the vulnerability-stress-competence model) by helping participants realize what can happen to them when they are not feeling well (i.e., how they see, hear, or feel things, and how these sensations are different when they are feeling well). These symptoms will be described in the next session as the expression of the interaction of participants' vulnerability and the stress they encounter.

The third goal is to continue separating thoughts from feelings. In the first activity on stress, physical, emotional, and cognitive symptoms of stress were presented separately. Here we also distinguish what is experienced in terms of thoughts and feelings, in order to prepare the participants for the ABC's of CBT for psychosis model presented in the next section.

Finally, the fourth goal is to enable the co-therapists to get access to the beliefs related to participants' symptoms. Some participants might have maintained their beliefs from when they were hospitalized and might appear to have very little insight into their experience, whereas others might not believe "as much," and others might have a quite sophisticated explanation for why they experienced such symptoms. Similarly, some participants might have adopted (or modified) a biological model to explain their experience, whereas others might believe that their hospitalization was due entirely to external circumstances (e.g., a bad batch of drugs), and others might feel they deserved to be persecuted because of past wrongdoings.

The session might also hint at some "core beliefs" held by some participants (such as "people are dangerous" or "I am a bad person"; see Chapter 2). The therapists should make sure to recall what was mentioned in this session because it will guide them for future sessions.

S-5 (Session 5): The Vulnerability-Stress-Competence Model

The vulnerability-stress-competence model is a central aspect of the group CBT for psychosis approach used here (as described in Chapter 2), but is also one of the most difficult sessions for the therapists to lead. In fact, seeing the pitfalls encountered and the mistakes made by various therapists in conducting this session, we have concentrated our efforts on simplifying the model, breaking it down into sections, and personalizing it in order for participants to understand its meaning and usefulness. Still, because participants can misunderstand some of the model's terms or concepts, therapists must be vigilant in verifying each participant's comprehension.

To start, the session summarizes what has been covered so far in terms of our knowledge regarding stress and how people react differently to stress. The concept of having a vulnerability or "sensitivity" to stress that is expressed differently for each person is then introduced. The understanding of the terms *vulnerability* and *sensitivity* needs to be verified. Some might perceive vulnerability as a weakness, whereas others might not

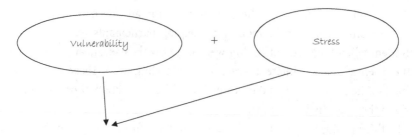

Depression (don't wish to do anything, stay in bed...)

FIGURE 7.2 Example of how to explain the vulnerability-stress-competence model.

have a clue about its meaning. Other expressions can be used instead, such as saying that someone is at "higher risk" or that something is "more likely to happen."

It is important to make sure that participants do not believe that having a vulnerability signifies that they are weak. The following explanation in the workbook describes how some people can be more vulnerable to gaining weight, developing diabetes, or having mental health problems. With some participants, this information can lead to tangential discussions regarding diabetes or weight gain; if that occurs, the therapists should bring participants back to the workbook and focus on mental health problems and protective factors. At this point, the participants will find there is a lot of information to take in; therefore, offering a concrete example is useful. Ideally, one of the therapists could use a personal example and write it on the flip chart as shown in Figure 7.2. Then the therapist could mention what is helpful when he or she starts having symptoms or not feeling well because of his or her vulnerability interacting with too much stress (Figure 7.3).

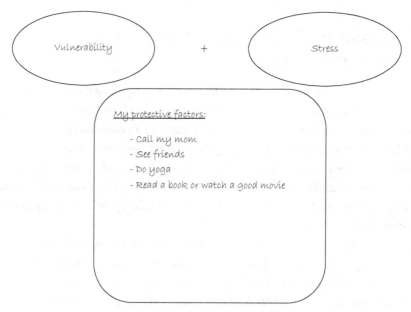

FIGURE 7.3 Continued example of how to explain the vulnerability-stress-competence model.

To make the model even clearer, we then ask the participants to give their personal examples, which we write on the same flip chart. Some participants might choose to say they are vulnerable to becoming "worried" or "scared" when in fact they have described delusions of paranoia and persecution in the previous session. That is fine—the therapist should write the terms used by participants. Regarding protective factors, some participants might mention substance abuse as their way of coping with stress. It is not the therapists' role to judge the answers, but it is possible to say, "Drugs or alcohol might help us relax at times. We will explore together in future sessions other coping strategies that might be more helpful in various situations."

Once this simplified and personalized vulnerability-stress-competence model has been discussed, we go over the "scientific" model presented in the workbook. We can use the protective factors mentioned by the participants to describe the various categories (e.g., "Calling my mom on the phone—that's family support"). We then ask everyone to take a few moments to write down their own protective factors according to the categories listed. The following definitions of each category are offered in the workbook to help participants decide how they should categorize their protective factors:

- **medication:** drugs prescribed by your doctor or psychiatrist . . . if you take them, what are they? Do you know what they are useful for?
- **social skills and competence:** abilities to talk to people, to ask for information or help when needed and to make friends.
- **coping skills, stress-management and self-esteem:** things you think about, say or do to feel better about yourself or to control your stress level or to diminish your symptoms (we will cover many in this group).
- **family and social support:** everyone who can offer support to you, counting family, friends, mental health staff, or others.

It is important for the therapists to make sure the participants understand how their protective factors can act as a shield against stressors in their lives. One of the goals of group CBT for psychosis is to help participants develop more and better protective factors. Not everyone will need to develop the same protective factors. Gaining an awareness of which protective factors the person already has and which categories might need to be developed further is an important first step toward building a greater sense of empowerment regarding one's mental health.

S-6 (Session 6): A Personal Goal

At first glance, session 6 appears quite different from the previous sessions because it presents the concept of goals and does not specifically relate to stress or to the vulnerability-stress-competence model. In individual therapy, clients usually begin with specific goals that they wish to accomplish in the therapy. In group therapy, given that we cannot adjust the therapy to accommodate each participant's goal, we propose instead that common themes can be helpful to everyone. Yet personal goal setting can act as a driving force for behavioral change. Therefore, we recommend that participants develop the habit of setting weekly goals that ideally, but not necessarily, are related to the content of the group sessions. At session 6, participants might wish to set as a goal to continue monitoring their stress levels or work on specific protective factors. Such goals would help integrate the content viewed so far, and participants could continue using the workbook and homework sheets to meet their goal.

The goals do not need to be exactly linked to the sessions. For instance, someone might specify as a goal that he or she wishes to be more assertive, and someone else might mention a goal of becoming a famous pastry chef. Those goals would be quite acceptable but would have to be broken down into smaller weekly goals. The acronym SMART, used for setting goals, can also be helpful for defining one's goals: S = specific ("being happy" is vague, whereas "doing at least one thing I like each day" is specific); M = measurable (so you know when you have reached the goal); A = attainable (because there is a plan, and steps are taken to meet the goal); R = realistic (becoming a musician may be realistic, whereas becoming a famous musician overnight is not); and T = timely (ideally can be attained in the near future). When working with people with psychosis, we often encounter two extremes: participants who have no goals and have difficulty finding something to strive for, and other participants who have what might appear to be grandiose goals. For the former, therapists will help them identify domains that are important to them (their health, friendships, schooling, and so forth) and will assist them in articulating both longer-term goals and smaller goals that could be accomplished within the next week. For the latter, it is important to not label the goals as unrealistic. For instance, the person who wishes to be a famous pastry chef might love baking but lack experience and training. The goal could be broken down into smaller steps, such as trying new recipes at home, looking into baking and pastry classes, and perhaps finding a part-time job in a pastry shop to see if it is really something the person would enjoy. No goal is judged as impossible or unrealistic, but when participants are helped to realize the steps needed to reach their goal, some might change their minds and choose another goal, whereas others might become even more motivated after seeing their dream is possible. It is important to remember that reaching one's goals is an essential step in building self-esteem. Having goals gives the person a sense of purpose and drive, whereas meeting a goal confers a feeling of accomplishment and competence. As mentioned previously, group CBT for psychosis aims at reducing distress by diminishing symptoms and strengthening protective factors, which include building strong self-esteem.

It is one thing to set goals; the participants must also try to meet those goals. To encourage participants, we have included the designation "partly met" in their weekly goal self-evaluation. Some participants become discouraged if they did not meet their goal, but a "partly met" goal can be praised and may lead to a "met" goal for the next week. Therapists are strongly encouraged to go over participants' homework at the beginning each session, including the "Goals of the Week" sheet every week. Participants can be advised to make their goals easier to meet or to choose goals that motivate them more, as needed.

Reviewing the First Section

Because session 6 is the last session of this section, we recommend a group overview of what has been accomplished so far. The therapists can ask what participants recall from previous sessions and what they wish to remember. If participants forget some elements, the therapists can add information regarding the themes covered and their purpose. Everyone should take some time to write down the elements they wish to remember and what they have learned. This overview not only allows participants to see the links between the different sessions and help them reflect on their experience; it also enables them to realize they have accomplished something—they completed the first section of the therapy.

Conclusion

The first section of the group CBT for psychosis aims to help people connect in a positive way while learning about important concepts that are not threatening or stigmatizing, such as stress. The sessions are planned to offer important tools without necessitating too much self-disclosure. After six sessions, participants typically have developed a strong alliance with the therapist and a good sense of cohesion with the group as a whole, enabling them to share their opinions and experiences more openly and to start working on more difficult themes. The next section introduces many of the most commonly used CBT for psychosis techniques and principles, which are always applied in a respectful and nonthreatening manner.

8

Testing Hypotheses and Looking for Alternatives (Sessions 7 to 12)

In this chapter we highlight the CBT for psychosis techniques needed for the second part of the therapy. We offer concrete examples of how to present the CBT model and techniques in a group setting, using short movies and neutral examples before tackling personal beliefs. Most techniques and activities start from the outside in, meaning that to avoid threatening participants, group members first practice the concepts with fictional examples before attempting to apply them to themselves.

T-1 (Session 7): The ABC's of CBT

At the start of each new section, it is important for the therapists to do a quick review of what was done previously (in a sentence or two) and present the objectives of the new section. We also recommend putting each session within the context of the module, mentioning that a quarter of the module has already been completed and that we are starting the second section. This helps participants not only to have a sense of what has been accomplished but also to keep in mind the time left in the group.

When presenting the A-B-C model, the goal is to help participants realize that it is not so much the event or situation that causes distress, but how they perceive the situation. It is helpful to use movie excerpts as illustrations. Different groups have used different movie excerpts, such as the scene in the film *Finding Nemo* in which two fish run into a shark and believe they will be eaten, only to find out the shark no longer eats fish. Some groups have used the film *American Beauty*—the scene in which a man believes he has seen his son have a homosexual interaction with the neighbor, whereas the son is actually helping the neighbor to roll a joint. The American insurance company Ameriquest created five brief, funny television commercials that can be found on

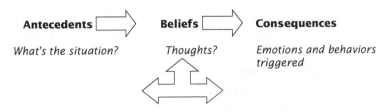

FIGURE 8.1 The A-B-C of CBT model.

YouTube and clearly demonstrate that what you see is not necessarily what is happening. The commercials all end with the reminder "Don't judge too quickly—we won't." Such movie excerpts and commercials make a strong point regarding the limitations of relying only on our perceptions when trying to understand a situation. Therapists need to take some time after viewing these examples to discuss with participants how we base our beliefs on our perceptions, and how thinking differently about a situation can lead to a different emotional reaction. Then the model is presented (Figure 8.1).

It is helpful to use the flip chart (Figure 8.2) and write on it the first fictional example from the workbook: "Two of my friends stop talking as soon as they see me." One of the therapists asks participants to take a moment to try to imagine what is going on, asks how they would be likely to feel and act in that situation, and instructs them to write it down in their workbook. Afterward, the therapist asks participants to share their answers and writes them down on the flip chart. Rarely do most participants mention the same

For each example listed, try to imagine yourself in that situation and describe what you would think and how you would feel and act.		
A *for* Antecedent What's the situation	**B** *for* Belief What do I think is going on?	**C** *for* consequence 1) How do I feel? 2) What do I want to do?
1- Two of my friends stop talking as soon as they see me		1) 2)
2- My new girl friend (or boy friend) seemed angry and canceled our date		1) 2)
3- The bus driver is looking at me funny		1) 2)
4- *Find your own example...*		1) 2)

FIGURE 8.2 Example of a group activity used to illustrate the A-B-C model while generating alternatives for beliefs.

answer, but it can happen that most answers are negative (e.g., "They are talking about me" or "They are hiding something from me"). In such cases, it is recommended that one of the therapists offer a very different answer, such as "Perhaps they wish to surprise me because my birthday is coming up" or "Perhaps they are discussing something very personal and do not wish to repeat the story."

The goal is to have a flip chart with different beliefs about the situation, which would lead to different emotional reactions and behaviors. The participants typically are quite surprised when they suddenly realize that people can experience the same event in very different ways. In fact, most tend to attribute their problems to situations rather than beliefs or perceptions, whereas this exercise clearly illustrates that it is the belief, not the situation, that makes the difference. The examples in the workbook use the same format and should be carried out in the same manner. The last one, however, asks for a personal example. Given time limits, therapists will rarely have enough time to go through more than one participant's personal example on the flip chart during the group, which is why we ask that everyone try to complete their personal example at home. It is important to review this example, as homework, at the beginning of the next session to verify if the A-B-C model was well understood and whether participants were able to apply it to their own experience.

T-2 (Session 8): Common Experiences

This session is about normalization. In the fourth session, participants had the chance to share their experience of their initial hospitalization or psychiatric consultation, but there was no emphasis on normalization. Here, examples are offered to help participants realize that unusual experiences can happen to most people when they are faced with unusual or extreme circumstances. Of course, having other people in the group with similar experiences can be normalizing in itself, but it is even more normalizing to realize that most people can hear voices or become fearful of others when they are sleep deprived or when mourning. The example of sensory deprivation used in the workbook can trigger various reactions depending on the group. Some might feel it is cruel to impose such experiments on people, others may be doubtful, whereas others will try to analyze why the brain reacts as it does. It is important not to get lost in details or stray off topic but instead to explain that people who have had voices or unusual thoughts do not have a "different brain," and that they are not "aliens" because all brains can trigger such unusual experiences. However, they might be more vulnerable to these experiences, especially when confronted with important stressors.

The following questions in the workbook relate to these experiences, which are divided into questions pertaining either to hallucinations or delusions, which in the workbook are called voices (or visions) and thoughts (fearful/persecution or powers/mission). Given that some participants might not have experienced one or the other, it is preferable to suggest that they answer both questions before sharing their answers. When reflecting on participants' answers, wording is important. For instance, the therapist might say, "So you *think* the FBI is after you because you have lied in the past" or "You *believe* God has chosen you to save our planet."

The last question refers back to the A-B-C model in a subtle way by asking participants to see the link between their thoughts or voices and behaviors. Although it is not clearly stated in the session, voices are treated as thoughts (or as the B in the A-B-C model) and will most often bring about a behavior. Not everyone will act on their belief or obey an order they were given by their voice. Some will refrain from doing things because of fear of increasing the frequency or intensity of the voices or fear of persecution. Therapists should acknowledge that some participants experience their voice(s) telling them to stop coming to the group, making participation difficult for them. Participants for whom this is the case will appreciate talking about it and receiving support from the group in order to attend in spite of the voice(s). Making the link between their unusual thoughts or voices and their behaviors will help participants realize the value of trying to see things differently and of perhaps changing their behaviors.

The end-of-session wrap-up should focus on the similarities in experiences between participants and how these experiences influence our behaviors. The following sessions aim to find different ways of looking at these experiences.

As mentioned previously, we encourage realistic goal setting every week. The homework is for participants to use their goal sheets, ideally integrating concepts or exercises presented so far such as monitoring their stress level and documenting (in a journal) their behaviors when experiencing specific thoughts or voices.

T-3 (Session 9): The Traffic Jam

This session aims at creating cognitive dissonance, which means bringing someone to the realization that he or she holds two opposite beliefs at the same time. Cognitive dissonance creates uneasiness, forcing the person to choose one of the beliefs and to reject the other. An example would be someone living in a suburb and working in the city who says that living in the suburb is great even though everyone knows there is significant road work being done at the time and it takes him more than an hour to drive into work. This person experiences cognitive dissonance between the thought "I love my house and my big yard in the suburb" and the thought "I hate the drive from the suburb into the city" and would therefore say that the traffic and road work are not that bad if you leave early for work. Cognitive dissonance is not always used in CBT for psychosis, but it can be particularly useful in a group context because it can help create a group consensus on a given topic. The idea in this session is to have everyone agree with the axiom "Any event can have several alternative explanations depending on the observer." If everyone agrees, then no one can also agree with the opposite: "Any event only has one explanation." In this session, participants will generate various explanations for situations in order to realize that alternative explanations can be found for most situations, especially when limited information is being offered. In a later session they will be asked to find alternative explanations for their own beliefs and will no longer be able to confirm that "only one explanation exists" for themselves, given they have agreed on the previous axiom.

This exercise is even more powerful when it is done in pairs. Participants can be asked to pair up and find at least two different answers for each question. The questions elicit alternative explanations but also different ways of seeking facts. The first question is quite neutral: "What causes a traffic jam?" But the following questions are more paranoia-inducing and require that participants work harder at finding alternatives. Indeed, finding more than one explanation for why people stare at you or why a pedestrian is forced into a car is more demanding than explaining a traffic jam. The co-therapists can assist the different pairs in the group in finding alternatives or means for checking the facts. We then recommend that the entire group gather and share their responses. As in session 7, it might be necessary for the therapists to suggest different answers (such as that the pedestrian is getting married and his friends are taking him out to a party).

Participants understand the idea of cognitive dissonance, and it can be surprising how well they integrate it in their own interventions. For instance, as mentioned in Chapter 4, participants in one of our groups were able to use cognitive dissonance to convince a group member not to commit suicide (saying that he believed in God and that God is against suicide). Also the peer pressure regarding cognitive dissonance has a strong impact: If we all agree that there is more than one way to see things, why would it be different for you?

The take-home message the therapists wish to convey is that there can be different explanations for most events, and unless we have all the facts, it is best to consider alternatives first.

T-4 (Session 10): How Not-to-Jump to Conclusions

As described in Chapter 2, it is well documented that people with psychosis, particularly with delusions, have a tendency to jump to conclusions, without gathering sufficient information prior to making a decision. The purpose of this session is to help participants think of facts whenever they are confronted with a story, somewhat like a detective inquiring about a crime. To start a session by asking participants to gather facts about their own beliefs would be too confrontational; we therefore propose scenarios that resemble the experience of someone with psychosis and ask participants to propose questions in order to gather facts. The idea is that they find pleasure in trying to find facts, and they apply this learning to their own lives. This activity works best when done in a role play. The following are a few tips to keep in mind when planning a role play:

- Announce that there will be a role play and indicate which character the therapist (or therapists) will play.
- Set the chairs for those doing the role play differently to clearly indicate they are not in the group but are acting.

- Use simple disguises, such as a scarf or a hat, that will be worn only during the role play, allowing participants to distinguish the "character" from the "therapist."
- Make sure to indicate when the role play is finished, remove the disguise, and bring the chairs back to their usual position.

These tips will ensure that participants do not confuse the role play with reality and that they will not become worried regarding the therapist's mental health. In this session, one of the therapists will role-play the first scenario (Andrew, the man who believes he was abducted by aliens), and the co-therapist will later role-play the second scenario (Sophie, who believes she can predict the future). Before starting the role play, we recommend that the therapist not doing the role play write down the questions a detective might use to find facts (the who, what, where, why, when) on the flip chart. Then participants are asked to address Andrew with questions that will help check the facts. The co-therapist writes down the answers on the flip chart while asking which fact the question is accessing. The therapist playing Andrew should not mention clear facts to prove his belief but can answer with vague answers or perceptions that he believes are true. Once most of the detective questions have been asked, the therapist asks the participants if they have sufficient facts to prove the story is true without a doubt. The answer should be no, which would lead the therapist to say that when there are not enough facts, it means that it could be true, or it could not be true, but we do not know for sure. The participants are then asked to try to come up with alternatives that could also explain Andrew's story.

Then the same exercise is repeated, with the therapist becoming Sophie and the co-therapist removing his "Andrew" persona and leading the activity. Of course, if two women lead the group, Andrew can become Andrea (or Sophie can become Steven if both therapists are men). A participant may find that the story is very close to his or her experience and could feel threatened by the exercise. Although we intentionally chose stories that we have often encountered, with the hope that participants will be able to apply the skills to their own experience, it is important to emphasize that it is not their story but the story of Andrew or Sophie. Participants might also have difficulties sticking to the detective clues and could start asking other kinds of questions (e.g., "How was the spaceship?" or "Were you scared?"). The co-therapist must guide them by asking whether or not the question really helps gather facts. Similarly, we do not ask participants if the story is true but rather if we have sufficient facts to know for certain. Therapists should ensure they exit the role play before reviewing what participants wish to remember about the session and describing the homework (using the ABC's of CBT for a personal distressing thought).

T-5 (Session 11): Considering Alternatives for My Own Beliefs

Session 11 is in many ways pivotal. Until now, many of the CBT techniques were used for external examples, with only small glimpses at using them for oneself. This session asks participants to use what they have learned so far in terms of the CBT model, seeking alternatives, checking facts, and applying these techniques to themselves. Furthermore, the aim is to help participants choose a belief that is as proximal as possible to their main issue or problem. The therapists need to keep in mind beliefs that were mentioned during the session, recalling participants' first consultation in psychiatry (session 4), as well as beliefs that were mentioned as still being present when the normalization activity took place (session 8), to help participants choose answers that will be central for them. Someone might mention that his distressing thought is that he has no friends. The same person might think that people are in fact jealous of his superpowers. In this case, focusing on the latter belief (jealousy) might be more central to his problems and could also partly explain his difficulty in making friends. It might be more difficult, and perhaps not warranted, to focus on the belief regarding superpowers given that it is a likely self-esteem enhancer, and attempting to create doubt could lead to resentment and frustration (see Chapter 2). The co-therapists might struggle to help participants find central beliefs to work on. It is not necessary that the beliefs be "core" beliefs, but as much as possible, they should be recurrent and often cause distress for the participant.

Questions 1 to 3 from the workbook can be answered alone, with the help of the co-therapists.

1. A thought or belief I hold that causes some stress and that often bothers me is:
2a. Because of this thought or belief, I often feel:
2b. Because of this thought or belief, I will:
3a. What are the facts that support my thought or belief? *(Name at least three)*
3b. Have all these facts been checked?

We recommend not asking participants to answer question 4 immediately ("Try finding at least one alternative explanation for each fact ") because it is very difficult for people to find alternatives for strongly held beliefs. In this activity, it is best to go through all the questions at once for each participant in turn; that makes it easier for the group members to suggest facts to consider investigating and to suggest alternatives. In fact, question 4 is best answered by the group members together. For some participants, therapists might need to repeat the axiom "Several possible explanations can be found for any given situation" (see session 9) in order to have participants agree to write down the alternative explanations offered by the group members. Some participants will be open to the suggestions and will participate willingly. Others will find this session extremely frustrating and will refuse to consider that their belief can be anything but the truth, refusing all potential alternative or fact-checking suggestions. In such cases, it is best not to insist and to ask, "If it is the case, how bad is it really?" to see if it might be possible to at least diminish the distress experienced. Someone might fear being kidnapped but has been living in the same apartment for years and taking the same routes to get home and has not yet been kidnapped; someone else might realize that although everyone talks negatively about him, they might not have much power over his life given he was able to obtain a job interview.

Although the goal of the activity is to induce doubt and help participants consider alternatives, when that is not possible, attempting to diminish distress by "dedramatizing" the belief could also be helpful. Although some participants might not be open to consider checking facts or to find alternatives for themselves, they could be very good at helping others. Even if some alternatives presented by participants may appear as irrational as the initial belief (e.g., "Are you sure it's the government? It could be the mafia"), the choice of alternatives is not important—to consider the alternative will induce doubt, regardless of the potential veracity. Typically, people who hold strong beliefs will not jump from one belief to another, but if they are able to simply consider the possibility that there could be an alternative, it will create doubt and could lead to changes in their emotional states and behaviors. As with the other activities, it is important to leave time for participants to reflect on the session and what they wish to remember about it.

T-6 (Session 12): Looking at Things From a Positive Perspective

The entire "T" section so far has been devoted to CBT for psychosis techniques. It comes somewhat as a surprise to finish the section with an activity that seems more related to self-esteem than to cognitions. This session actually does both. Session 11 might have been experienced as particularly difficult by some; proposing a session covering an important aspect of self-esteem will be welcomed by many. However, it is not only a "feel-good" session given that the concept of attributions is presented and can be linked to the A-B-C model of CBT, whereby some individuals might have a pattern of always perceiving events in a certain manner. This activity is greatly inspired by the positive psychology movement, particularly by Martin Seligman's *Learned Optimism* (2006), and focuses on helping people realize they might have tinted glasses (an attributional bias) that make them interpret situations in the same manner, regardless of the context.

Therapists might choose to start the session by placing a glass of water in the middle of the table and asking if the participants see it as half full or half empty. A discussion about optimism or pessimism can follow, prior to starting the activity. It also helps to copy the equations that are in the manual (positive things = outside attributions, positive things = self-attributions, etc.) and go over each one to make sure everyone understands before starting the activity per se. The word *attribution* might be difficult for some to comprehend; it might be useful to think of synonyms such as "who is responsible." As can be noticed, the attributions chosen in this activity pertain mostly to pessimism or optimism and not so much to paranoia. It is, however, possible that someone mentions always blaming others for all the harm that happens in his or her life and never attributing anything negative to him- or herself. In such cases, we recommend simply reflecting, without being confrontational, that when we believe that things are *always* a certain way, we most likely have tinted glasses that make us see things in only one way and that, in all likelihood and at least in some situations, there could be other ways of seeing things (i.e., alternative explanations).

Participants might have difficulty finding positive things that are related to their own actions. For instance, someone might mention being happy about an upcoming outing, but the outing is not linked to any form of achievement and is open to everyone. Someone else might mention winning a small sum of money at the lottery as something they are proud of, although such luck is not linked to any personal effort or achievement. Similarly, some participants might choose examples of negative outside attributions that could be considered inadequate or flawed. For example, a participant might mention having stolen something in a store, and it was a negative experience because he or she got caught. The therapists need to guide the participants in finding positive situations that they might have caused, and negative situations that appear accidental. The homework is to repeat the same exercise at home, using different examples.

Because half the sessions have now been completed, it is important to mention this in an appreciative tone, emphasizing the work accomplished so far. Therapists should ask participants if they recall what was discussed over the last six sessions and what they wish to remember (i.e., what is more relevant or important for them), while adding missing information and their own answers.

Conclusion

This second section of the therapy introduces most of the CBT for psychosis techniques that will be used until the end. Participants will be asked to continue applying them for themselves, as well for the others in the group. The group should have a solid identity during these sessions, having had the time to build a strong sense of cohesion. Participants should be staying longer for the socialization period than they did after earlier sessions. Most of the CBT for psychosis techniques presented so far have been linked to changing thoughts or beliefs; the next section will deal more with difficult emotions and problematic behaviors.

9

Drugs, Alcohol, and How I Feel (Sessions 13 to 18)

The third section of the workbook focuses on the emotional and behavioral manifestations of distress, as well as on self-esteem, and further develops the concept of coping strategies. Why discuss distress, specifically substance misuse and suicidal thoughts? These issues are not specific to individuals with psychosis, but they are prevalent in this population and all too often are addressed only when they become overly problematic. Clinicians can at times hold the false belief that CBT for psychosis should focus solely on psychotic symptoms. In fact, a good CBT for psychosis therapist will focus on distress, as well as on strengths and goals, which means the therapy will target not only psychotic symptoms but also other distressing emotions and behaviors. Similarly, the therapy should focus on the person's strengths, capacities, and goals that go beyond distress reduction.

This section of the module deals with distressing thoughts, behaviors, and emotions but also with positive and uplifting self-esteem activities. The self-esteem activities are intentionally presented before discussing the more difficult themes, namely, substance abuse, suicidal thoughts, sadness, and anger, in order to ensure that the participants have a positive view of themselves before exploring darker or more difficult aspects. If we keep the A-B-C model in mind, the previous section of the workbook targeted mostly the B, by helping participants understand their beliefs and introduce doubt, whereas this section focuses more on the C: emotional and behavioral consequences linked to distress. Some of the behaviors explored can also be understood as attempts at coping, some of them healthier than others. Healthy and often useful coping strategies will also be discussed and explored in the last section of the workbook.

D-1 (Session 13): Words That Describe Me

Given that this is the first session of the third section, the therapists should take a few moments to recall what has been accomplished so far and mention the objectives of this section. The purpose of the day's session should also be explained. It may seem obvious that to spend some time on positive qualities is a good idea even if the impact of such an activity might be less obvious. As mentioned previously, self-esteem is not a global concept and is developed through the building of different aspects or senses of self, such as the sense of security, sense of identity, sense of belonging, sense of direction, and sense of competence. The sense of identity implies knowing oneself, in terms of both limits and strengths. All too often, individuals who have gone through a life-changing experience such as a psychotic episode will describe themselves in pathological terms or will mention only their negative qualities when asked to describe themselves. Some will indeed struggle in this exercise to find more than two or three positive qualities.

The current session will demand a bit of preparation. It is recommended to have pages of the flip chart taped to the walls, with one page per participant (and one per therapist as well), with the names clearly indicated. This is a basic positive-quality self-esteem activity and should be done cheerfully; typically, it lifts spirits, and every participant leaves with a smile.

When starting the activity, the therapists should take the time to read (or ask a participant to read) each positive quality in the table out loud to verify that everyone understands its meaning. Then participants take a few moments to circle the qualities they feel they possess. The therapists should go around and make sure each participant has chosen at least three qualities but no more than six (we wish for them to pick their most central qualities). Then they are asked to transcribe these on their poster sheet on the wall. Each participant will then be asked to add one or two qualities to the poster sheets of the other participants. The therapists should do the activity as well and at the same time verify that the qualities added by the participants are just that: qualities. Given that they do not have to select qualities from the table, some participants will mention qualities that are superficial (e.g., nice hair) and are not as meaningful for the person receiving them as a quality linked to his or her behavior or personality.

Once the writing is done, each participant goes back to read what is now written on his or her poster sheet before starting the discussion. The discussion follows the typical format: Someone reads the first question, everyone takes a few seconds to jot down their answer, and people share their answers with the group. The idea behind this session is not only for participants to recognize their qualities but also to realize how they feel when they think about having these qualities. Most participants will be glowing, and some might show some disbelief when they realize that others in the group see qualities in themselves they had never acknowledged before. We wish to emphasize how we are too often reminded of what we do wrong and our negative sides, but we are rarely reminded of our good sides. Focusing on positive qualities and going back to them (keeping the list or poster sheet) can be helpful in periods of hardship. Participants are encouraged to keep their poster sheet with their positive qualities at home, where it is easily accessible. Make sure to allow participants a few minutes at the end to write down what they wish to remember from this session.

D-2 (Session 14): What I Value

This session continues with another self-esteem activity, this time focusing on values. Like the normalization activities presented earlier, this activity involves linking people together who share something similar—in this case, values. The idea is to create a sense of belonging, an important component of self-esteem, that is based not only on difficult experiences but also on something positive, namely, having similar perceptions of what is important in life. Although not everyone in the group will share the same values, many values will be shared by a few participants. Values guide a person's actions and goals and are therefore important to identify and to keep in mind. Although many values will be shared, some will not, and that is fine as well. As with all the activities in the workbook, there are no good or bad answers, and participants should not feel at odds with the others for having one or two values that might differ. Most values are, however, universal and will likely be shared by many members of the group. For instance, many participants will realize that they share the values of helping others or enjoying spending time alone. Others will realize that it is important for them to feel proud of themselves and also to maintain close family ties. We have included some values that might appear "materialistic," such as making money (many will indeed mention that money is important to them). The idea is not to judge or rank some values as being better than others but rather to help participants realize the values that are important for them.

The activity is quite straightforward: The participants take a few minutes to write down their answers, and the therapists count their hands and write on the board how many participants shared which values. A discussion follows about whether the participants feel they act in accordance with their values and how they do so. For those who wish they could act more in accordance with their values, the group can explore different ways this could be achieved.

This activity can also inspire goals for the goals of the week homework, particularly for participants who mention a value as extremely important but also indicate they are not doing enough in that domain.

D-3 (Session 15): Drugs and Alcohol: When, Where, and With Whom

This session is about developing insight into one's behaviors without prior judgment. Its focus is on helping participants understand the circumstances involved in their substance misuse. Often, participants will describe abusing drugs or alcohol without knowing why they did so at a certain time or in a certain context. They might realize that they abuse substances more when they are alone or when they experience peer pressure, or they might recognize that they are using these substances much more frequently than they initially thought. This realization can trigger, in some, feelings of worry regarding their substance use. Some participants might notice that they drink more when they are out in public, as a way of overcoming their shyness or social anxiety, whereas others might smoke marijuana more out of boredom, when they are alone at home. Drinking and substance misuse can be seen as coping mechanisms for participants facing difficult emotions or stressful situations. Other sessions will deal with healthier coping strategies; in this session, the therapists only need to help the participants realize why they are using.

It is possible that some participants avoid all drugs and alcohol and have never had a problem with these substances. Although it is unlikely that the entire group avoids all substances, given that close to 50% of individuals having experienced a psychotic episode will have had a substance misuse problem at one time or another, the activity might need to be modified to accommodate those without substance use problems. There are a few options, such as asking them to think about whether they have any addictive behavior (e.g., smoking cigarettes, overeating, gambling) and to answer the questions with that behavior in mind. Another option would be to think of people they know who might have addiction issues and offer their input from an observer's point of view.

In the rare case when no one in the group has any current issues with substances (ideally, the therapists should check one or two sessions before this session takes place to make adjustments if needed), the session could be skipped altogether, or the activity could be presented somewhat like a journal club where everyone discusses an article (written for laypeople) describing the link between cannabis use and psychosis, for example. The latter option has been tried before and was greatly appreciated by participants.

As for therapists, it is important not to self-disclose too much during the sessions on drugs and alcohol. Although therapists' participation in the group often involves giving personal examples, the participants should not have to worry about the therapists' current alcohol or drug use. If the therapists wish to share, they should mention experiences from their past, ideally not too extreme or problematic, rather than any current drinking or substance misuse.

As with all the sessions, make sure to keep a few minutes at the end for participants to write down what they wish to remember.

D-4 (Session 16): Their Effect on My Life

This session continues on the theme of substance misuse but looks at the effects of substances, both positive and negative. Many treatment manuals for people with mental illness focus only on the negative aspects of substance misuse and ignore the reasons that might bring someone to use, such as for relief from stress, for pleasure, for socialization, or for increased alertness. This session explores the short-term and long-term positive and negative effects of substance use. Some participants might feel that, other than feeling a bit slowed down the next day, they do not really have a problem with substance misuse, whereas others might realize that their substance abuse is having negative consequences in many areas of their lives.

The therapists should not suggest that everyone avoid substances but instead should help people gain insight into their behaviors and the consequences of these behaviors. Some participants might wish to boast about their varied substance misuse; this should be reframed with respect, emphasizing that no abused substance, no matter how enjoyable at first, is free of negative consequences. Even if physical or mental consequences are denied, most participants will agree that substance misuse is expensive and can have a detrimental impact on their budget.

A few suggestions are offered in question 4 regarding possible solutions if someone wishes to stop or diminish their substance misuse.

4. If I wanted to diminish or stop my alcohol or drug consumption, I could . . .

   ☐ A) change friends, if they were my drinking or drug buddies
   ☐ B) avoid hanging out at places where I would usually consume
   ☐ C) try other ways to make myself feel better (e.g., exercise, arts, movies, relaxation)
   ☐ D) learn to say NO and be assertive about what I want in life
   ☐ E) join a support group (live or internet) to help me quit
   ☐ F) find someone to talk to when I feel tempted or down
   ☐ G) do nothing, I don't drink or take drugs
   ☐ H) other:_____

For most individuals with a real substance misuse problem, however, specific services and therapies (above and beyond the group CBT for psychosis) are likely to be needed. Because the group CBT for psychosis manual cannot address this in depth, it is the therapists' role to ensure that those who might have specific needs are guided toward the best possible services. This means that the therapists should know where the participants could receive specialized substance misuse (or dual-disorder) services if needed, or at least make sure the participant's principal mental health worker can help with the referral. As mentioned earlier, the group CBT for psychosis manual was designed to cover many issues that are documented as central for people with psychosis and that can be at least partially targeted by CBT for psychosis techniques. As a consequence, some issues, namely, substance misuse, can be addressed only briefly.

At the end of the session, when all the questions have been discussed within the group, it is important to reflect on the two sessions on substance misuse and allow time for participants to write down what they wish to remember. The homework is to complete a "Goals of the Week" sheet and could be used for a goal linked to decreasing or changing substance misuse, if it applies. Otherwise, any goal linked with participants' recovery goals or to the previous sessions is recommended.

D-5 (Session 17): Feeling Down or Hopeless

This session deals with a very sensitive topic: suicide. Studies report that more than 40% of individuals who have been diagnosed with a psychotic disorder such as schizophrenia will attempt suicide at least once in their lifetime, and 5% will not survive (Palmer, Pankratz, & Bostwick, 2005). The subject of suicide can be difficult to address for therapists, but it is an essential one for participants. Because it is a delicate subject that might bring back intense emotions, the therapists need to make sure participants do not leave the session in a negative emotional state but instead are hopeful for the future.

In this session, hopelessness and suicidal thoughts (and behaviors) are discussed but from an external perspective at first (i.e., a role play). As mentioned previously, this indirect approach is used to introduce the topic delicately and to avoid forcing participants to discuss their own experience too quickly if they do not wish to.

One of the therapists will role-play the suicidal person (keeping in mind the rules for a good role play mentioned previously). After the therapist has set the tone by role-playing someone who is feeling hopeless, the co-therapist guides the participants by looking at the following questions in the workbook:

1. What <u>questions</u> might you ask that can make the person doubt that dying is the best choice? Go ahead, ask!

_____

_____

_____

2. What might you <u>say to convince</u> that person that suicide is not the solution? Try it!

_____

_____

_____

Participants are asked either to ask questions or to say something to the person in the role play to convince him or her that suicide is not an option. As the participants attempt to change the person's mind, the co-therapist can write their questions or comments, as well as the answers, on a flip chart.

Participants can also be guided toward using techniques and strategies used in previous sessions, such as checking the facts, seeking alternatives, self-esteem, normalization, and even cognitive dissonance (e.g., "If you believe that every cloud has a silver lining, then you can't be sure that your situation will never get better"). It is important that the therapist in the role play answers positively to the questions and comments by reconsidering his or her decision to commit suicide. The co-therapist wraps up by mentioning the techniques and strategies proposed by participants and asks the therapist in the role play to rejoin the group.

The next questions become more and more personal, starting with "What can someone do to get out of that feeling of hopelessness?" and following with the participants being asked if they have ever felt hopeless or suicidal and what they did to get better. Although an important part of the session is about sharing a difficult experience, the most important aspect is sharing and finding coping strategies to use when faced with hopelessness. The role play can be shortened if participants seem at ease in discussing the topic and suggesting techniques and strategies. Participants are likely to suggest useful strategies—the therapists only have to keep in mind the concepts and techniques used so far and suggest some strategies to the group that were not mentioned and ask for their opinions. It is important that participants leave the session feeling hopeful that, although such feelings can be painful, there are ways to overcome them. If the therapists feel that the morale is still low at the end of the session, they should make sure to ask participants to stay for the socialization period and discuss lighter subjects, or ask everyone to share a happy thought or even a joke.

D-6 (Session 18): Changing My Mood

This session deals with the negative emotions of sadness and anger. It may seem that many sessions are spent on issues that are not directly related to psychosis. In fact, the issues and emotions covered in the last few sessions all deal with very important and frequent emotions and issues that face many individuals with psychosis. Psychotic symptoms often fluctuate depending on how well someone can regulate these difficult emotions. Individuals with psychosis, even with nonaffective psychotic disorders, often struggle with periods of depression or intense frustration. These difficult and intense emotions may arise after the diagnosis of a psychotic disorder or following an injustice or stigma they have experienced, or they could be normal reactions to life events. This session does not attempt to understand the reasons behind these difficult emotions but instead focuses on coping strategies, particularly ones that peers have found work best for them.

The co-therapists are not asked to contribute much in terms of content during this session. Instead, their role is to facilitate the sharing of useful strategies for coping with difficult emotions. They can offer some personal coping strategies if they wish. Given that drugs and alcohol have been discussed previously, it is unlikely that participants will mention substance misuse as a good coping strategy here. Therapists might need to suggest alternatives if the coping strategies are not realistic (e.g., "Shop till you drop" can be hard on a limited budget) or if they are likely to cause more harm than good (e.g., "Punch the person who insulted you in the face"). Otherwise, the therapists are asked not to judge the suggested coping strategies, even if some might seem odd.

Participants are asked to take a few minutes to answer the first question on coping with sadness and to share their answer. We then ask participants to pick one strategy suggested by someone else that they would be willing to try. This session requires everyone to listen to others' suggestions in order to consider which ones might work best for them. The same process is used for the second question on anger. The homework of the day is for participants to try one of the strategies suggested by another participant during the next week and see if it works for them.

Given that this is the last session of the section, it is important not only to take a few moments for participants to note what they wish to remember from the session but also to review the earlier sessions within this section. Participants can recall the striking moments they remember, and the therapists can also recall topics that have been discussed previously but were not mentioned by participants. In planning ahead, the therapists should ask participants to dress comfortably for the next session because a relaxation technique will be practiced. The therapists should also make sure that they have mats available. It should also be mentioned that because only six more sessions are left, participants should start thinking about what kind of graduation they would like to celebrate the end of the group.

Conclusion

This chapter has described the third section of the workbook, which asks for participants to use many of the CBT for psychosis techniques described in the previous section. These sessions cover challenging themes, such as substance misuse, hopelessness, and difficult emotions, as well as positive themes linked to self-esteem and values. The following section of the workbook continues to use the CBT for psychosis techniques that have already been presented but focuses more specifically on coping strategies and relapse prevention.

10

Coping and Competence (Sessions 19 to 24)

This chapter describes the last section of the workbook. It is titled "Coping and Competence" because it aims to explore the adoption of new and useful coping strategies for different contexts. Coping is not only about making it through a stressful situation but also implies using daily strategies that can help prevent greater difficulties in the long run. The focus is also on preventing mental illness relapse by encouraging insight into one's warning signs of relapse and concentrating on protective factors and recognizing which coping strategies are most useful for which difficulties or symptoms.

As with all sessions, it is important first to review the homework—in this case, trying a new coping strategy for difficult emotions proposed by a peer. The therapists can then make the link with the current section and explain how additional coping strategies for dealing with stress, emotions, or symptoms will be explored for new contexts, as mentioned in the learning objectives.

It is essential to remind the participants that there are only six more sessions and take a few minutes to discuss ideas for the end-of-group celebration. This celebration is an important event and should be planned carefully. Many participants might have had difficulty in the past finishing a project or obtaining their high school diploma; thus, to have completed the 24 sessions of the group is an even greater achievement for them. Also, spending 24 sessions together, over the course of 3 or 6 months, creates a strong sense of belonging and cohesion that can be hard to leave behind. Groups that have not carefully planned their ending can bring about feelings of loss and sadness in participants. The clinical team or primary mental health worker for each participant should be made aware that the group is coming to an end and that new projects need to be planned and started soon. This is why there is an emphasis on things to continue working on and celebrating an accomplishment (rather than mourning the loss of the group). Similar to a school graduation, the end-of-group graduation should include receiving a diploma (a template is offered in the Appendix 2) and can involve, depending on the available budget and the participants' preferences, a potluck meal where everyone brings something to share, a restaurant dinner, a delivery meal (such as pizza), fun snacks, decorations, music (commercial or performed by participants or therapists); it can involve just the group or also invited guests. The discussion around the graduation party can take place over more than one session, but it needs to be started at this point. Take only a few minutes to discuss the graduation before starting the session.

C-1 (Session 19): Relief From Stress

This is a very popular session with participants because it offers a simple, easy-to-use, and effective relaxation strategy that can be applied in various situations. As with most sessions, a participant should volunteer to read the top of the page in the workbook, and then someone else reads the rest of the page. The idea is to help participants realize that stress is not to be avoided at all costs; some stress is needed in order to perform and achieve goals in life. One of the therapists can copy the figure from the workbook and explain it on a flip chart (Figure 10.1).

It is important to explain that when stress becomes extreme, we need to find ways to calm down to avoid becoming overwhelmed and incapacitated. The relaxation activity proposed here serves this purpose.

Various relaxation techniques exist, with some focusing more on specific muscles, others on thoughts or mantras, and others on energy levels (chakras). We intentionally chose a relaxation technique that is quite concrete, requiring individuals to concentrate on their breathing by asking them to breathe in a different way than usual. The relaxation activity is influenced by Buddhist mindfulness practices, in which thoughts that appear during the relaxation technique are not judged or resisted but rather are acknowledged and let go. During this activity, participants may repeat the word *Shavasan* (the name of a yoga relaxation posture) or the word *relax*.

Slowly and with a calm, steady voice, one of the co-therapists reads the Shavasan exercise. Therapists need to make sure participants are at ease, the room is well prepared for the activity (no noise, dimmed lights), and everyone feels safe. Although it is recommended

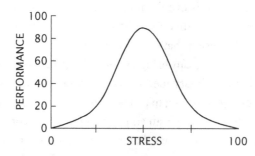

FIGURE 10.1 Cognitive and behavioral coping strategies

that participants close their eyes and lie down on a mat during this exercise, some participants prefer to do the exercise sitting down, and some might even prefer to their eyes open and sit with their back to the wall. The activity should last at least 20 minutes, but no more than 35 minutes, to get the full benefits and have time to reflect on the experience. Make sure to leave enough time for participants to re-emerge after the activity is completed, slowly bringing them back into the group and turning the lights back on. The participants and co-therapists may share what they liked or disliked about the exercise, how it can affect their stress level (in their body, mind, emotions), and whether they think they would use it again. It is possible to memorize the technique and use it, in a briefer version or sitting down, in various situations such as on the bus or in a classroom.

C-2 (Session 20): Dealing With Symptoms

This session is challenging for therapists and participants because it involves recalling central symptoms (delusions and voices) and distressing thoughts and thinking back to the coping strategies that have helped in the past. The session aims to explore new and diverse coping strategies, based on the cognitive and behavioral techniques experienced so far. It is important to acknowledge what already works (i.e., the coping strategies that participants have been using so far to cope with their symptoms, psychotic or other). The idea is not to dismiss participants' current coping strategies but to expand their repertoire to include more strategies that they could use in different situations or contexts. Listening to loud music might help someone with his voices, but it might not be possible to use this strategy if the voices are bothersome at work, for instance.

The group begins with questions 1 and 2 from the workbook:

1. When I experience the symptom

_____

what usually helps me is

_____

if that doesn't work, I try

_____

if things seem to be getting worse I will

_____

_____

_____

One thing that doesn't help me is

_____

_____

_____

2. When I start having the disturbing thought of

_____

_____

what usually helps me is

_____

if that doesn't work, I try

_____

if things seem to be getting worse I will

_____

_____

One thing that doesn't help me is

_____

_____

The co-therapists help each participant individually, making sure that all partici-pants write down an important symptom (most often a psychotic symptom) and distress-ing thought (psychotic or not) and ensure that they have identified the most frequently used coping strategies for dealing with the symptoms or thoughts. The questions also introduce the idea of a gradient of severity, with the participant needing to choose what to do if one coping strategy does not work or if the symptoms appear to worsen. The questions may help some participants realize that they often use the same coping strate-gies regardless of the severity of their symptoms and even if things do not improve.

We also ask what participants feel does not work for them. This last question is important given that participants have likely attempted to use several coping strategies in the past and might even have been told to try specific strategies by their parents or a mental health worker, and they already know what does not help them. Then, take a few minutes to share with the group the answers to questions 1 and 2.

THOUGHTS	BEHAVIORS
☐ concentrate on the type of voice, tone, male or female, etc.	☐ take a hot bath or shower
☐ think of something positive or nice about myself	☐ have a massage
☐ try to think of why I'm thinking this, what are the antecedents, what's the situation and what are the consequences of my thoughts on how I feel and behave	☐ try relaxing techniques
	☐ listen to music
	☐ watch television
	☐ take walk
	☐ exercise(sport)
☐ try to assess if I'm perceiving things right by checking for evidence	☐ humming or singing
	☐ speak to myself
☐ remind myself that even if my thoughts are scary, the situation is not really that bad ao dangerous	☐ call a friend to talk
	☐ go see a movie
	☐ read a book or magazine
☐ Try to see things from a positive perspective by changing the attributions I make	☐ play a game
	☐ go on the internet
☐ forgive myself for wrong doing	☐ clean my room
☐ give myself pats on the back to encourage myself	☐ go check for evidencefor my beleifs
	☐ ask people I trust if my beleifs, make sense and if they can hear the same voices
☐ tell myself that I have resources I can use to overcome my symptoms	☐ write diary of my emotions and daily thoughts
☐ accept myself with strengths and challenges	☐ call my physician, case-manager or nurse to make an appointment
☐ try thinking and considering every possible alternative for my belief	☐ take my meds regularly
☐ try thinking of something else	☐ participate to group meetings or activities
	☐ do something with my hands (crafts, drawings...)

FIGURE 10.2 The stress-performance curve.

Question 3 involves looking at a long list of cognitive and behavioral coping strategies (Figure 10.2). Participants are asked to check all the strategies they have tried that have worked (at least somewhat); to cross out those they have tried that have not worked, or those they would never try (e.g., some people will never clean their room as a coping strategy); and to circle those strategies that could appeal to them. They may also add strategies suggested by other participants in the group that are not on the list. In this activity, it is vital for participants to consider their own preferences, and also to "get out of their comfort zone" and try new strategies they might not have considered before. Even if someone mentions not liking exercise, he or she might be surprised at the benefits of going for an energetic walk when distressing thoughts are present. The homework in this session is central—participants are asked to try at least one new coping strategy during the week.

C-3 (Session 21): Available Resources

The previous sessions as well as this session all involve the development of protective factors. Coping strategies are essential when dealing with stress, difficult emotions, and symptoms, but so is a good support network. In this session, the focus is on support—not only emotional support but also informational and material support. Participants might have one or two people they can count on in times of need but could come up with more names if they really think about who could help them with a specific need. As with coping strategies, the goal is to expand participants' support networks by helping them identify who could offer a specific type of support. Some community organizations and mental health professionals are well equipped to offer information regarding symptoms and medication, whereas other individuals, such as family and friends, might be better suited to offer emotional support. Similarly, one needs to think carefully about whom to ask for material support, depending on what kind is needed (e.g., a parent might lend money, but asking a friend for money could harm the friendship).

Therapists should ask participants to answer one question at a time and share their answers with the group. It is not necessary to write a name in each category; some categories could also have more than one name. Some participants might feel they do not have many names to write down, either because they have a restricted support network or because they cannot think of anyone; if this happens, the other participants and the therapists may be able to make suggestions. It often happens that participants offer their own names and phone numbers for someone else in the group who needs a support person.

Besides the list of individuals who might be part of a support network, this question involves choosing a close, trustworthy person to share symptoms and coping strategies with. This person needs to care enough about the participant to accept being part of his or her plan for staying well (i.e., the relapse prevention plan detailed in session 23).

The therapists should bring a list of community resources available in the area to offer the participants after the discussion on their personal support networks. Various community organizations can offer different types of support, such as housing, work, affordable food, and community shared cooking, as well as mental health services (crisis phone lines, drop-in services, support groups, etc.). The therapists should take a few minutes to go over the list with the participants.

The homework is in continuity with the session, in that participants are asked to write down the name and phone number for each support person they have identified on the appropriate sheet in the workbook. The next time they need a specific type of support, they can easily access their support person by referring to this list.

C-4 (Session 22): My Strengths, Protective Factors, and Challenges

This session brings back the vulnerability-stress-competence model, but this time participants are asked to reflect on what has changed in their model since the beginning of the group. Throughout the group, participants have learned to see and act differently in order to cope with stress, their emotions, and their symptoms. They have unveiled some of their strengths and positive qualities and have also discovered that some problems or issues might need continuous effort to solve or improve. In individual CBT for psychosis, one's formulation changes over time as goals are met or problems are resolved. Similarly, the vulnerability-stress-competence model changes as participants develop new protective factors and are better able to cope with their symptoms and the stress in their lives.

The therapists should ask participants to answer one question at a time and share their answers with the group. The first two questions are as follows:

1. What do you consider your strengths to be?
2. What are your protective factors?

For these questions, participants can mention strengths or protective factors they already had at the beginning of the group, but they should be encouraged to try to think of new ones that might have developed throughout the sessions. The following questions are asked next:

3. What are your problems or difficulties?
4. How will you go about overcoming these problems?

For these questions, too, some problems might still need to be worked on, but participants should be able to suggest solutions or strategies. The group is not meant as an end to all problems—participants will need to continue working on some issues, and it is important for them to realize that it is OK to still have issues and to persevere in their attempts to improve their situation.

The final question in this activity ("In what do you consider having improved yourself?) refers to the sense of competence, the last stage in the development of healthy self-esteem. Throughout the group, participants have set goals for themselves, tried new behaviors or ways of thinking, and most likely improved in ways they might not have expected. The improvements do not need to be directly related to symptoms or stress per se. For instance, one participant might mention being better at interacting with others and making friends, whereas someone else might find it easier to ask for help or avoid abusing drugs. The vulnerability-stress-competence model is presented once more, to give participants an opportunity to master it. Many participants in past studies have mentioned that this model had helped them feel more empowered and in control of their mental health.

As with all the earlier sessions, a few minutes are planned at the end for participants to reflect on what they wish to remember from the session. The homework here is not directly related to the current session but is essential for the next session, which involves developing a staying-well plan. The homework involves rating one of the "Effects of Stress" checklists to the Group CBT for psychosis workbook (Appendix 1) while keeping in mind how things were immediately before the person needed to seek psychiatric help. This will help determine warning signs in the next session.

C-5 (Session 23): Coping My Own Way

"Coping my own way" is essentially a staying-well plan or a relapse prevention plan worded positively. In this penultimate session, the participants have a pretty good idea of what works or does not work for them and under what circumstances. This session provides a synthesis of that information. It allows participants to reflect on their best coping skills to stay well daily, to help them meet their goals and stay well when faced with adversity and stress. By having all these coping strategies written down in the same place, and by sharing this information with a trusted person, participants are more likely to use the strategies. In a few months' time, or in times of stress, participants might forget the coping skills they have explored and found helpful during the group, relying only on the strategies they have used the longest. The "coping my own way" staying-well plan is a document they can refer back to and that a trusted friend or family member can also refer to, if needed.

As with most sessions, the participants will share reading the heading, description, and questions of the activity. The first two questions refer to cognitive ("I will tell myself . . .") and behavioral ("I will do . . .") coping strategies to stay well daily. These daily strategies should include elements of a healthy lifestyle as well as a positive outlook on life. Of course, the answers will originate from the participants, but therapists can also suggest some ideas. It is well known that people with a mental illness who maintain a healthy lifestyle by sleeping enough hours at night, eating healthy and regular meals, exercising, and having fulfilling activities are more likely to stay well than those who have less healthy pleasures and structure in their lives. Similarly, beliefs about being able to stay well and the person's self-perceptions also greatly influence recovery and staying well. It is also useful to help participants phrase their sentences positively. For example, it is best for them to write, "I will tell myself I am strong and capable" instead of "I will avoid putting myself down." Participants should write down more than one element for each question. These can include some of the coping strategies discussed previously, other protective factors (social support, medication, stress management, etc.), or any other element that will most likely contribute to their recovery. The therapists act as guides in this session, helping participants find their answers and encouraging them to add to their answers.

Questions 3 and 4 ask about the cognitive and behavioral strategies needed to meet one's goals:

3. In order to meet my long-term goals while staying well I must tell myself:
4. In order to meet my long-term goals while staying well I must (do):

Although it is likely that the strategies used daily to stay well might also help someone meet their goals, it is important to avoid overlap and to find answers that are more specific to the person's goals. Participants have filled out "Goals of the Week" sheets throughout the duration of the group and have a pretty clear idea of what is important to them and what they wish to accomplish. They might, however, need a bit of help in finding which coping skills or thoughts and behaviors might help them in meeting those goals. The therapists can suggest thoughts linked to perseverance, positive qualities, and strengths or setting smaller goals, making schedules, planning ahead, and so forth.

Question 5 ("I know things start going wrong before my symptoms get worse when I am experiencing the following") refers to warning signs or symptoms persons might experience when they feel overwhelmed by stress before they see their symptoms worsening. To answer this question, participants are asked to use their last homework assignment, in which they completed an "Effects of Stress" checklist on how they were doing physically, psychologically, and emotionally before they last sought psychiatric help. If some participants did not do their homework, ask them to take a few minutes now to complete it (by going back to pages 10 to 13). The answers should be copied onto the lines for question 5. Typical answers are linked to changes in sleep, poor hygiene, racing thoughts, trouble concentrating, fear, guilt, isolation, or lack of motivation.

Questions 6 and 7 refer to the warning signs written down for the previous question:

6. When things aren't going so well, either because I'm experiencing high levels of stress, my symptoms are getting worse or I'm very depressed, I should tell myself:
7. When things aren't going so well, either because I'm experiencing high levels of stress, my symptoms are getting worse or I'm very depressed, I should (do):

The coping strategies named here should be those that are the most effective for each person in order to avoid a relapse. For instance, if a participant realizes that it really helps her to check the facts with a friend when she fears she is being followed, this should be written down. Someone else might write that a slight change in medication (to help him sleep) would work, as well as reading to diminish the voices. The participants can go back to sessions 18 through 20 to remind themselves of the new strategies they have found particularly helpful when faced with stress, symptoms, or difficult emotions. It is essential that participants write down only strategies they are likely to use, those they have tried, and those that were successful for them. Of course, it is possible that participants are influenced by each other and wish to add elements to their answers following the discussion, which is also fine as long as they are convinced they are likely to use that strategy when needed.

Finally, participants are asked to share their staying-well plan with someone they trust and see regularly. Normally, they should have written down who that person is during session 21. It would be best if this person were not a mental health professional, given that professionals can change jobs and are not always available. A close friend or a family member who is involved in the participant's life is a good option. Sharing the plan ensures that someone else can help the participant realize when things are not going well and help him or her adhere to the staying-well plan if the person's resolve is sliding or bad habits are coming back. The trusted person can also remind the participant of coping strategies he or she had tried before that had worked. Having a trusted person who also knows the staying-well plan serves as extra insurance in case the participant needs reminders or support.

The group should take time to reflect on the activity, its purpose, and the future use of the staying-well plan. During the socialization period, therapists should also discuss last-minute details about the graduation party that will happen either immediately after the following session or on another day (in the same week). Although it is great when there are enough funds to pay for a restaurant meal for the group or order pizza, a large budget is not necessary. Some popcorn, decorations, music (chosen by participants), and juice or soft drinks can suffice. Therapists should make sure to print out a diploma before the party for each participant who is present.

C-6 (Session 24): Review of the Module

This is it: the last session. Therapists should take the time to remind the participants of everything they have accomplished in the past 23 sessions, asking if they recall all the different themes covered and adding some details as needed.

The session is a reflection on each person's experience, what each of them liked, disliked, and learned during the group. The questions can be asked one at a time, to allow for discussion and avoid long silences. As with most sessions, the therapists may also share their own answers. The therapists should take notes, especially about elements that were most liked or disliked and what participants found most useful. These answers can guide the therapists in their next group by helping them identify where they might make small changes or focus more on certain elements.

The only question in this activity that is not about the past (i.e., what has been experienced during the sessions) is question 8 ("What are you going to continue working on in the near future?"). This question is purposely asked at the end to help participants realize that although they have completed the module, they should continue having goals and values to guide their behaviors. Often, when the group ends, participants feel ready to embark on another big project, such as going back to school or work, or starting another therapeutic activity that earlier might have seemed too demanding. The group CBT for psychosis can act as a steppingstone for participants. It is therefore important that the clinical team be ready to help participants who have recently finished the group to meet their other recovery goals.

Graduation Party

We have mentioned the importance of celebrating the end of the group at various points in the previous chapters. This moment is experienced as an achievement for many participants, some of whom might not have completed a project in years, and it is therefore essential to honor it by making it special. The therapists who conducted the group need to be present, and they should have organized this enjoyable moment with the entire group. The celebration can take place immediately after the last session or later in the same week. Diplomas should be given for each participant, even those who missed some sessions (see the example in the Appendix 2. Of course, some participants will likely be sad about the group coming to an end, having created close bonds with the participants and therapists. Therapists need to acknowledge this loss while also focusing on the future and the projects that the participants wish to accomplish.

Conclusion

Chapters 7 through 10 have offered a detailed description of how to conduct group CBT for psychosis by following our workbook. Of course, there are other models of group CBT for psychosis, as described in Chapter 3, but we have chosen to present in detail our approach, which we not only developed but have repeatedly tested and validated. The following chapters offer other useful tools, such as measures that can be used to assess the impact of the group or how to deal with difficult clients or situations when running the group, as well as a brief overview of other CBT-derived group approaches for people with psychosis or their family members.

Measuring Change

The success of cognitive behavioral therapy in general, as well as CBT for psychosis, stems in great part from demonstrating changes in symptoms over time, with measures showing improvements between pretherapy and both post-therapy and follow-up. This chapter proposes measures that can be used quickly and efficiently in a clinical setting to demonstrate the impact of the group CBT for psychosis. Measures specific to CBT for psychosis such as the CHOICE (CHoice of Outcome In Cbt for psychosEs), as well as measures of concepts that have shown improvements following CBT for psychosis, such as symptoms, self-esteem, coping skills, social support, self-stigma, and social functioning, are described. Other measures of interest to assessing processes in therapy, such as alliance with therapists, group cohesion, participation within the group, and measures of treatment fidelity or therapist competence, are also suggested.

Why Measure?

In times of economic austerity, health services, including mental health services, need to justify their expenses and use of staff. Although offering services in groups can appeal to managers seeking to diminish the cost of treatments, clinicians should still demonstrate the usefulness of their group intervention to maintain it as part of the services offered. It is also rewarding for clinicians and participants to "empirically" observe how the group might have brought about different changes in the person's life. The results should not be reserved only for managers but could be shared individually with participants when meeting with their lead clinician. Measuring the impact of a group does not need to be a lengthy process; many validated measures are easy to administer and to interpret. The following measures proposed here have been used in various studies and various clinical settings. We have intentionally chosen measures that do not necessitate lengthy training or supervision or that can be administered only by professionals with specific credentials.

CHOICE: A Measure of Client Perception

One interesting measure that has been developed especially for CBT for psychosis is the CHoice of Outcome In Cbt for psychosEs (CHOICE; Greenwood et al., 2010). This consumer-developed measure assesses various therapeutic goals that a participant might have upon starting CBT for psychosis. The measure consists of 24 items that measure both one's current assessment of various domains, such as symptoms, self-confidence, and coping with distress, and one's satisfaction with each domain. Although the various items can simply be added together to yield an overall recovery score, clinically it can be of interest to look at changes over each domain in terms of clients' current assessment of themselves and in terms of their satisfaction with each domain. We recommended having participants fill out the questionnaire prior to starting the first group session and having them complete it again after the last group session.

The questionnaire is currently available on the website https://www.sussex.ac.uk/webteam/gateway/file.php?name=choicefull.pdf&site=75 or by writing directly to the first author.

Outcomes

Various outcomes can be expected from participating in group CBT for psychosis. Among these, the most explored have been changes in symptoms, with more recent studies also documenting changes in psychosocial constructs such as self-esteem, coping, social support, social functioning, or self-stigma.

Symptom Measures

The symptom measures most often used in CBT for psychosis studies are semistructured interviews conducted by psychiatrists or psychologists, such as the Brief Psychiatric Rating Scale (BPRS; Ventura et al., 1993), the Positive and Negative Symptom Scale (PANSS; Kay, Fiszbein, & Opler, 1987), and the Psychotic Symptoms Rating Scales (PSYRATS; Drake, Haddock, Tarrier, Bentall, & Lewis, 2007). Although these measures are well validated and offer relevant information in terms of symptom severity, frequency, and impact on life, they necessitate extensive training prior to using them with clients.

Another option for clinicians wishing to determine if the group CBT for psychosis had an impact on their clients' symptoms is to use a self-report measure such as the Brief Symptom Inventory (BSI; Derogatis & Melisaratos, 1983). The BSI, which has been validated across various populations and languages, measures distress as well as psychiatric symptoms in less than 15 minutes. It consists of 53 items and measures nine dimensions: somatization (7 items), obsessions and compulsions (6 items), interpersonal sensitivity (4 items), depression (6 items), anxiety (6 items), hostility (5 items), phobic anxiety (5 items), paranoid ideation (5 items), and psychoticism (5 items). The items can also be added in three different ways to offer three global indices: Global Severity Index (GSI: the sum of all items, essentially a total distress score), Positive Symptom Total (PST: the number of symptoms reported by the client), and Positive Symptom Distress Index (GSI divided by PST, or the equivalent of a total severity of symptoms score). The BSI instrument is not freely available but can be purchased in a paper or computer version, with or without the scoring system, through Pearson (www.pearsonclinical.com).

Self-Esteem

Improving self-esteem and maintaining a healthy self-esteem are essential aspects of group CBT for psychosis. Although various self-esteem measures exist, some are not very sensitive to change over time and are therefore not recommended as an outcome measure. The Rosenberg Self-Esteem Scale (Rosenberg, 1965), for instance, includes only 10 items and is quick to administer, but it was designed to assess global and stable trait self-esteem—meaning that it is not meant to assess subtle changes in self-perception over time. A good measure to determine if the group CBT for psychosis led to changes in self-esteem is the Self-Esteem Rating Scale—Short Form (Lecomte, Corbiere, & Laisné, 2006). This 20-item self-report measure is derived from Nugent and Thomas's (1993) longer version of the tool and offers both a positive (10 items) and a negative (10 items) self-esteem scale and has demonstrated sensitivity to change over time. Individuals with psychiatric disorders can at times see only one aspect of their self-esteem change over time, either the positive or the negative, which is why these two scales are relevant and often more useful than the total score (sum of both scales). Given that our team validated the scale, it can be found in the Appendix 5. The items with an asterisk need to be added together to form the negative self-esteem scale. The negative score should be multiplied by −1, meaning that the score should be less than 0 (therefore, a bigger score indicates worse negative self-esteem). The other 10 items should be added together to create the positive scale. A total score can be obtained by adding both scales together. The total score is always inferior to the positive score because the negative score is less than 0.

Coping Skills

There exist several measures of coping skills in the literature, often theoretically based and proposing various subscales according to each theory. For instance, Lazarus and Folkman (1984) developed the Ways of Coping Checklist (WCCL) to distinguish two main coping strategies: problem-solving, or one's attempts to change the stressful situation; and emotion-focused, or one's efforts to self-regulate emotions when change does not appear possible. Edwards and Baglioni's (1993) Cybernetic Coping Scale (CCS) sees stress as an interaction between a desired state and one's actual state, with coping being one's attempt to diminish the negative impact of this discrepancy on one's well-being. Other measures have also been developed, namely, the Coping Inventory for Stressful Situations (CISS;

Endler & Parker, 1990), the COPE (Carver, Scheier, & Weintraub, 1989) and Brief COPE (Carver, 1997), and the Coping Strategies Inventory (CSI; Tobin, Holroyd, Reynolds, & Wigal, 1989). A review of coping measures (Guppy et al., 2004) criticizes most of them in terms of poor psychometric properties, with many of the theoretically derived subscales not matching the data (and therefore suggesting poor construct validity and often borderline reliability). One potential explanation for the less than adequate psychometric properties of some coping measures could be the number of subscales. Although these subscales might make sense theoretically, they are often too numerous and contain only a few items each (e.g., the Brief COPE has 28 items but 14 subscales).

One coping measure that is recommended for both its psychometric properties and its usefulness with various clinical populations is the CCS (Edwards & Baglioni, 1993). Although the authors recommended the 20-item version over the original 40-item version, a more recent 15-item self-report version proves to be even superior in terms of psychometric properties (Guppy et al., 2004). This briefer version maintains the five coping dimensions developed by the original authors, namely, changing the situation, accommodation, devaluation, avoidance, and symptom reduction. Each dimension contains three items. For clinicians, it is interesting to document if participants in the group CBT for psychosis use more "active" coping strategies after taking part in the group, such as changing the situation, accommodation, or symptom reduction, or if they continue essentially using "passive" strategies such as avoidance and devaluation when confronted with stress. The instrument can be obtained by writing to the author, Julian A. Edwards (email on publication: j.a.edwards@mdx.ac.uk).

Social Support

As with coping, social support has also benefited from the development of several measures over the years (Gottlieb & Bergen, 2010). Some measures focus more on the number of contacts per week a person has, whereas others measure more broadly whether the person has someone who can offer a specific type of support. The Multidimensional Scale of Perceived Social Support (Zimet, Dahlem, Zimet, & Farley, 1988), for instance, is a one-dimension, 12-item, self-report instrument that assesses how one perceives the support offered by friends, family, and a significant other. The measure does not take long to answer and is offered at no cost at http://www.yorku.ca/rokada/psyctest/socsupp.pdf.

However, if one is interested in specific aspects of social support, an interesting measure is the Social Provisions Scale (SPS; Cutrona & Russell, 1987). This not only measures support received but also reciprocity in support (i.e., support given). The SPS includes 24 items that tap into six types of provisions available from the general social network (4 items for each dimension), including reliable alliance (practical help), guidance (informational support), attachment (emotional support), social integration (belonging to a group of similar peers), reassurance of worth (esteem support), and opportunity to provide nurturance (providing support to others). We recommend this latter measure to assess specific changes in support following the group CBT for psychosis, given that often only one or two dimensions of social support will change over the course of a brief intervention such as group CBT for psychosis. Please be aware that some items will need to be recoded before being added to create the subscales (i.e., 1 = 4, 2 = 3, 3 = 2, and 4 = 1). The authors ask that an email be sent to them to obtain a copy of the measure at drussell@iastate.edu.

Social Functioning

Social functioning includes everything needed to live successfully in today's society, such as independent living skills (cooking, cleaning, hygiene, etc.), engaging in positive relationships with family and friends (social skills), and abilities at school and work (Lecomte, Corbière, & Briand, 2008; Lin, Wood, & Yung, 2013). It should not be confused with quality of life, which reflects satisfaction with various aspects of one's life. For instance, people might improve in terms of social functioning but see their quality of life decreasing because they have increased expectations. Group CBT for psychosis does not directly target social functioning, but it could help improve some aspects because of the strong focus on meeting one's goals and also because of the social context in which the group takes place. However, the measure of social functioning is problematic because it is affected by the age of the person, the opportunities available to him or her, and the time that the measure was devised (e.g., expectations of roles change over time, particularly for women). Specific domains of social functioning could however change depending on the type of group, and the potential social goals of the group members. For instance, there is less likelihood of changes in family dynamics or in employment behaviors during group CBT for psychosis, but friendships and social activities may change.

A clinician-rated single-score general scale such as the Global Assessment of Functioning (GAF; APA, 1987) or the Social and Occupational Functioning Assessment Scale (SOFAS; APA, 1994) would not be likely to detect change over time in social functioning for participants in the group CBT for psychosis.

Similarly, the most often cited comprehensive measure of social functioning for people with mental illness, the Social Functioning Scale (SFS; Birchwood, Smith, Cochrane, & Wetton, 1990), is also unlikely to change over the course of group CBT for psychosis. However, some of its subscales linked to socializing might change slightly. The SFS includes seven subscales: withdrawal/social engagement (e.g., time spent alone, social avoidance: 5 items), interpersonal communication (number of friends, quality of communication: 5 items), independence-performance (performance of independent living skills: 13 items), independence-competence (perceived ability in independent living skills: 13 items), recreation (engagement in hobbies, pastimes: 15 items), prosocial (engagement in social activities, sports: 23 items), and employment/occupation (engagement in productive employment or structured daily activities: 5 items). Each subscale has a different number of items and is rated in various ways (Likert scales, checklists, ratings from 0 to 100, yes/no answers, numeric answers [e.g., number of friends]). The SFS can be answered in self-report but is somewhat easier to administer with the help of a clinician or assistant. The scoring can be a bit tricky but is explained in the guidelines offered with the instrument. The SFS and guidelines can be obtained by contacting the author, Max Birchwood (last documented email: M.J.Birchwood@warwick.ac.uk).

A recent social functioning measure that was designed specifically for individuals with early psychosis (i.e., young individuals who might socialize both via technology and in person) is the First Episode Social Functioning Scale (FESFS; Lecomte, Corbière, et al., 2014). The FESFS measures both perceived ability and actual frequency of performance of behavior for each dimension and has demonstrated adequate psychometric properties. The measure consists of nine dimensions: friendships and social activities, independent living skills, interacting with people, family, intimacy, relationships and social activities at work, work abilities, relationships and social activities at school, and educational abilities. Each domain offers two scores (ability and performance) and can be obtained by simply adding the scores of the items under each heading. There is no total score given that the instrument taps into very different aspects of social functioning. In our own study, we have seen significant changes in some of the subscales following group CBT for psychosis (Lecomte, Corbière, et al., 2014). The measure is available in the Appendix 6.

Self-Stigma

Although few studies have assessed the impact of group CBT for psychosis on self-stigma, it is foreseeable that the group could have an impact on the participant's acceptance and endorsement of stigmatizing views regarding mental illness, mainly because of the normalization that takes place during the sessions. Given that people who are less affected by self-stigma tend to lead more productive lives and develop better social networks, measuring changes in self-stigma can be of interest. A few measures of internalized stigma have been developed over the years, but the most widely used and validated one is the Internalized Stigma of Mental Illness scale (ISMI; Ritsher, Otilingam, & Grajales, 2003). In addition to producing an overall score, the ISMI contains five subscales: alienation, stereotype endorsement, discrimination experience, social withdrawal, and stigma resistance. The alienation subscale is a measure of the subjective experience of being less than a full member of society. The stereotype endorsement subscale measures the degree to which the respondent agrees with common stereotypes about people with mental illness. The discrimination experience subscale measures the respondent's perception of current treatment by others. The social withdrawal subscale measures avoidance of social situations because of mental illness. And the stigma resistance subscale is reverse-scored and reflects the experience of not being affected by internalized stigma. Both the total and subscale scores are calculated as a mean, with possible total and subscale scores ranging from 1 to 4 and larger scores indicating greater self-stigma. The original version consists of 29 items, but a more recent 10-item version, with apparently adequate psychometric properties, is also available (Boyd, Emerald, Otilingam, & Peters, 2014). The ISMI (short or long) can be obtained by contacting the first author, Jennifer E. Boyd (last documented email: jennifer.boyd@va.gov), with the recent short version also being available in the published article (Boyd et al., 2014).

Process Measures

Clinicians will often not take the time to assess elements that might influence the success of a therapy, such as the participants' actual participation in each session, the alliance between therapist and client, or the group cohesion between the participants in a group. Yet these concepts can help explain why some participants benefit more than others. Those who have avoided interacting during the group sessions and have more trouble developing an alliance (or with whom the therapists have more trouble developing an alliance) might not invest as much in the group CBT for psychosis and are less likely to see strong improvements during the course of the therapy. Assessing these concepts during the course of the therapy can help the therapists make adjustments if needed, discuss the issues with the participants, or at least better understand the outcomes.

The Group CBT Participation Rating Scale

The group CBT participation rating scale (Leclerc, 1998) is easy to use after each session and allows the therapists to reflect on the session and recollect specific details regarding each group member's participation. The scale, referred to briefly in Chapter 5, covers various behaviors linked to participation, such as verbally intervening, maintaining eye contact, helping others, asking questions, paying attention, and socializing, as well as two elements that are coded negatively (i.e., their scores are subtracted from the total): disruptive behavior and confusion. Very often, therapists will notice changes in the participation rating scale for each participant over time. These can also be graphed and shown to participants in the group (using the average score for the group) or individually, and shared alone with each participant. See the Appendix 4 for the scale and its scoring system.

The QuickLL

The QuickLL (Lecomte, Spidel, & Leclerc, 2005) can be considered a snapshot of how the participants currently perceive themselves. The QuickLL contains 14 questions asking the participant to rate "right now" how he or she perceives the group, the other participants, the therapists, and his or her own self-esteem, optimism, and current symptoms on a 3-point scale. The measure takes less than 2 minutes to answer and helps participants become more mindful of how they are at the moment. The results can also be charted for each participant (and shared individually with them). Our own studies suggest that a very instable alliance as measured by the QuickLL, for instance, is linked to fewer improvements in symptomatic outcomes (Lecomte, Leclerc, Wykes, Nicole, & Abdel Baki, 2014), and that participants' perception of the usefulness of the group becomes more positive as their symptoms improve during the sessions (Lecomte, Leclerc, et al., 2014). The QuickLL is available in the Appendix 7.

The Working Alliance Inventory

The Working Alliance Inventory (WAI; Horvath & Greenberg, 1989) is the most studied and validated measure of therapeutic alliance. The original version consists of 36 items rated on a 7-point Likert scale and offers three scales: goal, bond, and task, as well as a total score. The measure offers two parallel versions: one for the client who rates his therapist, and one for the therapist who rates his client. The goal subscale assesses if one feels they are both working toward similar goals, the bond subscale reflects more the appreciation of the relationship and trust, and the task subscale measures how well both agree on the tasks (e.g., homework) involved in the therapy. A briefer version (12 items) of the WAI has been validated and has strong psychometric properties while maintaining all three dimensions (Hatcher & Gillaspy, 2006). The WAI can be obtained for free on its specific website: http://wai.profhorvath.com/.

The Cohesion Scale

The concept of group cohesion has been measured in various ways over the years, with some researchers focusing more on attractiveness of the group members, conflict resolution, or the alliance between members. According to Burlingame McClendon, and Alonso (2011), most measures will assess aspects of cohesion pertaining to the *structure* of the relationship (i.e., the direction and function of the relationship, including perceived warmth, competence, and tasks in the group) or will focus on the *quality* of the relationship (i.e., belonging, acceptance, alliance, group climate). Few measures include both aspects, and fewer still assess perceptions linked to individuals in the group, the therapists, the group as a whole. The Cohesion Questionnaire (Piper, Marrache, Lacroix, Richardson, & Jones, 1983) is such a tool. It was developed to assess cohesion according to three angles: the participant rating the group as a whole (i.e., the other participants), the participant rating the therapists, and the therapist rating the participant as a group member. The questionnaire assesses various aspects of group cohesion, namely, regarding seeing positive qualities in group members or therapists, feeling a personal compatibility with group members or therapists, and appreciating the therapists' leadership (or appreciating the participant's role in the group). Each item is rated on a 7-point Likert scale. Although the measure taps into various aspects of cohesion, it is fairly quick to use. It is possible to obtain a copy and guidelines for using this tool by contacting John Ogrodniczuk at ogrodnic@mail.ubc.ca.

Measures of Treatment Fidelity

Treatment fidelity measures for CBT for psychosis are scarce, and even fewer measures exist for group CBT for psychosis. However, some measures were designed for general individual CBT and can help verify if the most essential aspects of CBT are respected. Among these, we find the Cognitive Therapy Rating Scale (CTRS; Young & Beck, 1980), which we have used in a slightly modified version for group CBT for psychosis. The measure allows an external rater, using audio or video material, to rate on a scale of 0 to 6 the degree to which the therapist performs on general therapeutic elements, as well as more specific CBT techniques and conceptualizations. The scale is available online, along with the guidebook, at the Beck Institute website (http://www.beckinstitute.org). The CTRS has been modified by Haddock et al. (2001) to include different anchor points and more guidelines linked to CBT for psychosis (called the CTS-Psy). It is scarcely used because the anchor points are not always logically scaled (i.e., a higher score does not always represent better mastery of the skill or domain).

Another tool is the Cognitive Therapy Scale-Revised (CTS-R; James, Blackburn, Garland, & Armstrong, 2001). The scale resembles the original CTRS in assessing both general therapeutic skills and more specific CBT domains, but it involves rating 17 different aspects and therefore takes longer to use. It is, however, considered somewhat of a gold standard measure in many training settings and could be useful to clinicians wishing to verify if they are following the CBT model and philosophy. It is also available online and, like the CTRS, is not specific to people with psychosis and not adapted to the group setting. Both measures have been used to assess therapist competence, but they actually are measures of treatment fidelity. In fact, a therapist can obtain a high rating, indicating that he or she is using CBT in a "textbook" fashion, but nevertheless not adapt flexibly to the client's needs and demands (see Chapter 13 for more details).

One group measure that is interesting to determine group therapy treatment fidelity, although it is not specifically related to CBT, is the Group Psychotherapy Intervention Rating Scale (GPIRS). This scale, translated from Dutch into English (Chapman, Baker, Porter, Thayer, & Burlingame, 2010), assesses how therapists ensure important aspects of group psychotherapy, namely, maintaining the group structure, facilitating verbal interactions, and facilitating and maintaining a therapeutic emotional climate. The measure is somewhat long (consisting of 48 items, some of which are not applicable at each session), but it is a good tool for group therapists who wish to assess their general group therapy skills.

Conclusion

This chapter addressed the relevance of using measures to determine outcomes of the group CBT for psychosis. To measure outcomes, it is best to use the same measure before and after treatment, and ideally also at one follow-up time, such as 3 to 6 months after the end of the group. Some measures of outcomes have been proposed, although many others are available. The measures suggested here are ones that we have used ourselves; other clinicians and researchers could propose other measures that are also well validated and interesting. It is important, as much as possible, to opt for measures that are easy to administer, are fairly brief, and have been previously validated and published. We have also proposed other measures that can be of interest, such as process measures and measures of treatment fidelity. Although these measures will not help convince a service manager to keep offering group CBT for psychosis, they can be useful for clinicians in terms of understanding what is happening in the group and for evaluating their own therapeutic skills.

Obstacles to Group CBT for Psychosis

Various obstacles can be encountered in group CBT for psychosis, either before, during, or even after the therapy. Some of these obstacles are setting-specific, such as lack of support from management; others are more therapist-related (e.g., feeling incompetent, not getting along with the co-therapist) or client-related (e.g., participants missing sessions, difficult clients). This chapter covers the solutions to these obstacles and challenges.

Obstacles Linked to Team Resistance

Most often clinical administrators are enthusiastic about group provision of treatment. The financial argument is strong: More clients can be seen at the same time. Group interventions that are brief and supported by empirical results are even more appealing. However, clinicians who are used to working with individual clients might not be as enthusiastic at changing their therapeutic way of working. A top-down management approach in which new groups are imposed on clinicians is likely to backfire and result in resistance, especially if the clinicians do not feel respected in their role, do not see the value of the group, or do not believe they possess the needed skills to conduct the proposed group.

The following are potential signs of resistance:

- Few clinicians volunteering to run the group (or a therapist having difficulty finding a co-therapist)
- Absence of referrals of participants to the group
- Indirect attempts at boycotting the group (e.g., scheduling other activities for the participants at the same time as the group)
- Perceiving participant change stemming from the group in a negative way

Solutions

First and foremost, it is important that the clinicians see the value of the proposed group, so the introduction to the group needs to be persuasive. Clinicians with no group experience or with little CBT for psychosis experience will need to receive training and supervision; ideally, they should conduct a group with a more experienced group therapist (described in more detail later) to help them become sufficiently competent to run a CBT for psychosis group. Change that is introduced slowly is typically easier to accept—for instance, running an initial group with enthusiastic clinicians and sharing the experience with the other clinicians will help increase the group's popularity within the team. This sharing of the group experience will also enable all the clinicians to understand what is being worked on and will help them see change in their clients, such as increased assertiveness or expressing more goals and demands (signs of increased self-esteem and empowerment), in a more positive light. Furthermore, not everyone should be asked to run groups. Clinicians who do not possess the necessary skills and/or are resistant to working in a group should also have a valued role in the team and the clinic. It is important that group CBT for psychosis be presented as a complement or supplement to other services but also as an essential part of a comprehensive service.

Scheduling and Budget Considerations

Although inpatient settings can usually find a slot during the day for their group, groups with outpatients might need to be scheduled in the evening, especially if some participants attend school or work during the day. However, most clinicians in outpatient settings also work during the day, for instance, from 9:00 a.m. to 5:00 p.m. Changing clinicians' schedules can initially seem difficult for clinic directors, especially if proposing a group implies changes in caseloads, changes in schedules or pay (having clinicians start their days later, accumulate extra hours worked, or get paid for overtime), changes in vacation times (to ensure both co-therapists are available for the duration of the group), or security issues (such as in an office that typically is closed at night). All these scheduling considerations need to be thought through before the first group is offered, but they are much easier to plan for future groups.

Another important consideration is linked to the budget. Groups are not expensive given that two therapists see many clients at once, but they typically run better if a small budget is allocated to the group. This budget enables group therapists to provide snacks and refreshments (or at least coffee or tea), offer a treat or meal at the graduation party, and pay for bus passes for participants who need them. Some clinic directors or managers might not consider that coffee or a snack is necessary, or that participants should be offered bus tickets, but these small expenditures can significantly improve attendance and help participants feel that the group is considered worthy by the clinic. Therapists asking for a small budget for the group might have to "sell" the importance of such a budget, justifying the advantages and showing that the group will be more successful if such expenditures are allowed.

Obstacle: Therapists Lacking Confidence in Running the Group

After having read this book or having received a workshop on group CBT for psychosis, many therapists can initially feel very enthusiastic about running their first group, but they might also feel worried or anxious on the days preceding the first group, doubting their ability to conduct the group. This nervousness is quite understandable, especially for therapists with limited group experience, but should not be a deterrent.

Solutions

When therapists are describing normalization, participants usually will be very understanding, even happy, to hear therapists mention that it is their first time conducting the CBT for psychosis group. As mentioned previously, it is helpful for novice therapists to have their initial group experience with a co-therapist who has some group experience, even if it was not specific to running a CBT for psychosis group. The workbook offers a useful structure and guide for beginning therapists to rely on. The therapists' confidence will increase as the group evolves and participants develop a sense of group cohesion and successfully start applying the techniques and strategies discussed in the group to their daily lives. The therapists will also feel more competent if they carefully review the content of each session prior to conducting it and also take some time to plan the sessions together before each group.

Obstacle: Difficulties Working in Co-therapy

The biggest therapist-related obstacle is often difficulties between co-therapists. Some therapists will naturally work well together, creating a fruitful and enjoyable collaboration. Others will not get along or may have such different values or therapeutic styles that working together is a weekly struggle. For instance, if a group is run by an optimistic therapist and co-led by a therapist who is negative, holds stigmatizing views, or does not truly believe in recovery, conflicts between therapists will likely emerge. A co-therapist who is passive, one who takes no initiative, or, at the opposite extreme, one who wants to run the show alone, barely allowing anyone else to intervene, can also be very difficult to work with.

Solutions: Choosing the Right Co-therapist and Getting Supervision

We mentioned the importance of the choice of the co-therapist in chapter 6, but we want to emphasize the importance of making a careful selection. Future group therapists should meet prior to starting the group so they can discuss their style, their beliefs about recovery, and their experiences with clients. Casual discussions about difficult clients or past group experiences can help therapists realize if they both hold similar views.

For example, one group co-therapist with experience in running groups and with skills exhibited during role plays could not let go of using medical vocabulary and constantly spoke about participants' illnesses, diagnoses, and psychiatric symptoms. Her inability to use the CBT framework and our nonmedical terminology would have become clear in a casual lunch meeting with the co-therapist, along with the right set of questions.

Expert Supervision

At times, it might not be possible to choose another co-therapist, either because of lack of personnel or because someone was hired specifically for that position. In such cases, when problems appear, supervision is the best solution. Ideally, the supervisor should be someone from outside the setting who has experience in group CBT for psychosis. Our team, for instance, has given supervision on numerous occasions, either regularly or sporadically, in person, over the phone, or via a videoconferencing online program such as Skype. Some settings do not have the resources or access to someone sufficiently qualified to offer such expert supervision, but other supervision experts could identify the issues between the co-therapists and offer appropriate help.

Peer-to-Peer Supervision

We often recommend peer-to-peer group supervision when several clinicians in a setting have been trained in group CBT for psychosis (e.g., have attended one of our workshops). In such settings, the therapists running the group either show videos of parts of sessions or describe how the group is doing and present some problems they have encountered. The peers then offer constructive feedback and, based on their recollection of the workshop and/or on their own group CBT for psychosis experience, they can suggest ways to overcome these difficulties. It can be a bit intimidating at first to use peer-to-peer supervision, but this feeling will quickly dissipate if this practice becomes part of the clinic's functioning (e.g., once every 2 weeks, clinicians have lunch together and discuss the ongoing groups). The basic rules of peer-to-peer supervision are as follows:

- Always offer positive feedback first.
- Ask relevant questions.
- Propose potential solutions with tact, to avoid humiliating the therapists being supervised.

Clinicians should always keep in mind that one day they might be the ones who will need supervision; a constructive and positive approach to giving feedback is always preferable to confrontation.

We have found that this peer-to-peer formula works well, particularly when paired with occasional refresher workshops or sporadic external supervision. For instance, some clinical settings have asked for a 1-day workshop on specific questions 1 year after the initial workshop, and others have asked for a 2-hour consultation to be reassured in their supervision and group processes. We realize that people are more accustomed to being supervised by "experts," and to supervise each other can be unsettling, partly because they are unsure of their own competence in running the CBT for psychosis group. We recommend that mental health workers recently trained in group CBT for psychosis quickly start running their first CBT for psychosis group, using the structured workbook and their basic knowledge and taking the time to thoroughly prepare themselves. True competence develops only with experience, self-reflection, integration of feedback, and learning from both successes and mistakes. The same guidelines apply for supervision, with the added importance of accepting that running CBT groups for psychosis might not be for everyone.

After attending a workshop (or when reading this book), mental health clinicians are typically able to recognize if they have the necessary skills to run group CBT for psychosis. (In Chapter 13, we present these essential skills as falling within three categories: *know* [basic knowledge of CBT for psychosis, *know-how* [understanding of group processes and abilities in maximizing them, and *know-how-to-be* [appropriate role and attitudes].) Some clinicians might not feel competent enough to run a group but might still be able to offer constructive feedback, especially regarding dealing with difficult clients.

Dealing With Difficult Participants

Although the vast majority of groups run smoothly, at times therapists might run into difficulties with specific participants, particularly those who do not attend regularly or those who exhibit challenging behaviors or attitudes during the group sessions. The following discussion is not exhaustive but covers some of the most frequent participant problems that can be encountered when running a group CBT for psychosis.

Attendance problems have been alluded to in Chapter 6 and can be linked to motivational problems (i.e., negative symptoms of schizophrenia), low expectations regarding the usefulness of group CBT for psychosis, cognitive problems (i.e., forgetting), daily stressors, or even changes in the weather. For those who might miss sessions frequently, therapists need to address the problem with the participants in order to find potential solutions.

Some potential solutions to attendance problems involve calling the participants a few hours before the group or the night before, having someone in their environment remind them or even drive them to the group, and suggesting to participants that they use the group as support for their daily stressors. Encouraging attendance by mentioning that their presence was missed and that others asked about them also works.

Depending on the therapists' experience and ease with specific client profiles, and also depending on the other group members, some participants can at times be experienced as rather challenging. The following is a nonexhaustive list of types of participants who can be experienced as difficult, along with suggestions for how to cope with them:

- The monopolizer: This participant tends to dominate the discussions, always has something to say, and will want the group to spend most of its time on his or her personal problems.
    - Solution: The difficult task for the therapists is to repeatedly interrupt this participant to allow others to speak. Because it was mentioned in the rules at the first session that everyone should have time to speak, most monopolizers will not be offended by the interruptions. Another option is to refer to an element mentioned by the participant and use it to ask a question of the other participants. This allows the participant to feel that what he or she was talking about has value while allowing others to participate. However, if this behavior occurs at every session, it might be necessary for the therapists to speak with the participant alone with a reminder of the rules and goals of the group and also to make sure he or she accepts that the group is based on everyone's participation. Some participants, for instance, those with comorbid personality disorders, may have trouble accepting not being the center of attention and might decide to drop out of the group after a few sessions.
- The mute: This participant is the opposite of the monopolizer and does not talk at all. Although most extremely shy individuals will refuse to participate or will come to only one session, some participants may attend the group diligently but not share their thoughts or answers and will at best answer in one or two words. The reasons for the muteness can be numerous: The person may not feel sure that the group is safe, may fear being judged, or may be experiencing symptoms (catatonia) or side effects of medication (feeling slow). This type of participant can be a challenge for therapists trying to find ways to engage him or her.
    - Solution: One suggestion is to engage the participant physically, such as by asking him or her to write on the flip chart. Therapists can also use various strategies to increase the participant's self-confidence by asking easy questions and emphasizing small accomplishments. Positive reinforcements, either verbal (e.g., thanking the person for contributing) or nonverbal (e.g., a warm smile when the person enters the group), can help engage the mute participant. If the silence lasts, the therapists should speak alone with the participant to better understand the issues at play. As mentioned previously, at times we have encountered participants who were mute for many sessions but suddenly became quite verbal once they realized the group was safe and that no one would judge them.
- The delinquent: This type of participant tends to brag about mischief, mentioning wrongdoings with pride and speaking of drug abuse and violence in positive terms. At times, he or she may swear and use inappropriate language. Depending on the group

member, this participant can intimidate others, even creating fear. The delinquent could also negatively influence other participants.

- Solution: The therapists need to be vigilant, interrupting off-topic discussions, reframing inappropriate language as disrespectful, and reminding the participant of the rules as needed. At times, when an angry outburst occurs or insults are spoken, it is necessary for one of the therapists to leave the group with the participant to discuss what is going on. Both therapists can also meet with him or her alone after the group to ensure that these behaviors will not reoccur. At all times, it is important that the therapists not respond aggressively to this type of participant. Our experience encourages us to avoid excluding participants based on occasional inappropriate behavior, preferring to limit the damage by helping the participant respect the group and participate positively. In fact, focusing on the participant's strengths and positive behaviors and qualities can shift him or her back to a healthier discourse and enable the group to continue discussing the day's theme in a respectful, enjoyable climate.

- The clown: The participant who acts like a clown, most likely to avoid speaking of personal issues, can disrupt the group by turning everything into a joke. The clown can make others laugh but at times can also infuriate participants who wish to gain as much as possible from the group experience.
  - Solution: To avoid humiliating this participant, it is important not to confront him or her directly in front of the other group members. Instead, the therapists should take him or her aside, before or after a session, to address the problem.

- The court order: Participants who are mandated by court order (such as clients receiving treatment in a forensic facility or prison) to receive group CBT for psychosis can be particularly difficult to engage. They not only have been forced to attend, and therefore have no intrinsic motivation, but also are aware of the absence of confidentiality surrounding all clinical interventions in such settings. For instance, a participant will not wish to disclose hearing voices if he or she knows that the information will be written in his or her file. The judge, having access to the file and knowing the participant still presents with psychiatric symptoms, could refuse a leave or a reduced sentence.
  - Solution: Unless the group therapists manage to find a way to limit the information going into the file and offer the group partial confidentiality, it is extremely difficult to conduct a real group CBT for psychosis in such forensic settings. With participants refusing to disclose personal information, the therapists can at best only deliver psychoeducation about CBT for psychosis.

- The very symptomatic: Some participants will wish to participate in the group but will be struggling with severe symptoms, especially in inpatient settings. Some might be constantly interacting with their hallucinations, trying to push them away, or mumbling to themselves throughout the session.

- Solution: Previously, we have provided examples of how these participants can still benefit from the group and should not be excluded if they can tolerate the group and are motivated to attend. We have, in fact, offered a briefer version of our group CBT for psychosis in short-term inpatient settings, using smaller groups (four to five participants), three times per week for a total of 16 sessions (see Appendix 3 for the list of the 16 sessions used). Although group CBT for psychosis includes concepts that might be difficult for some participants to grasp, most will retain information that they believe will be useful. However, when only one or two participants in a group struggle with severe symptoms, they might be more difficult to engage, might tend to keep to themselves, and could therefore be a challenge for group therapists. Ideally, someone who is too confused and disorganized could be screened prior to the beginning of the group and not be invited to join if most of the other participants are well stabilized. A group could, however, include a few very symptomatic participants. In such cases, the therapists need to use more repetition and need to encourage and thank group members for their participation even if their answers might sometimes be off. The other participants will most often be very empathic and understanding of the person who is more symptomatic and will wish to keep him or her in the group.

- The confronter: At times, group therapists might encounter a participant who seems to seek confrontation with the therapists, asking trick questions or constantly contradicting them. By doing so, the confronter seems to want to unsettle the therapists, make them lose credibility in front of the other participants, or make them look incompetent. In fact, these behaviors can be seen as attempts to avoid change and to escape truly engaging in the group and the activity.

  - Solution: Therapists should avoid answering trick questions directly and instead bounce them back to the participant or refer them to the group members, asking them to answer the questions or give their opinions. A confronter who does not succeed in discrediting the therapists, and who furthermore starts feeling isolated, being the only one who opposes an activity, will likely join the ranks and stop confronting the therapists (or will drop out of the group).

- The narcissist: This type of participant clearly mentions from the start that he or she is superior to the other participants, discredits their input, and suggests that his or her answers and opinions are more worthy. This superior attitude can be detrimental to group cohesion, setting the narcissist apart from the others.

  - Solution: The best way to deal with a narcissist within the group is to first validate the participant and then help him or her realize that everyone can have different perceptions or opinions and that none are "better" than others. The "Yes . . . but" formulation typically works well: "Yes, it is possible that for you exercising is the best way to deal with stress, but for others in the group, other strategies might be preferred." At times it can also be useful to reinforce the rules, stating, "No answer is ever judged as good or bad" and reminding the participant that the goal is not to find the best answer but to find what will work best for each person in the group.

- The withdrawn: A participant who is withdrawn can appear bored or simply not invested. Therapists might wonder why this participant continues to attend the group because he or she does not seem interested, is hard to engage, and seems pessimistic about the group's potential for providing any help. Yet the fact that this participant attends can be a sign that he or she has some form of hope that the group will be helpful.
  - Solution: Therapists need to reach out more to these participants by questioning them about their past experiences, helping them see the value of their knowledge and answers, and exploring with them their personal goals. Eventually, the withdrawn participant might perceive him- or herself as useful to the group, and in turn see the group as useful.
- The expert: This participant might have past experiences in therapy or in groups, or might have read various self-help books and will make sure everyone in the group is aware of his or her "expertise." The expert will often intervene, sharing his or her "vast" knowledge and trying to replace the therapists. The problem with the expert is that he or she will be convinced of holding valuable knowledge but very often will be "off," making wrong assumptions or mixing up unrelated concepts.
  - Solution: Although it may be tempting for the therapists to discredit or ridicule the expert, it is best to validate the participant's quest for knowledge and to emphasize the need for the group to stick to the concepts and examples proposed in the workbook so that everyone can benefit. If the expert wishes to share other readings or past therapeutic experiences, the socialization period might be a better time for him or her to do so.
- The "overly emotional": This participant has trouble controlling his or her emotional outbursts, resulting in periods of intense crying or dramatic expressions of joy or anger. At first, participants and therapists might feel uncomfortable witnessing the participant's tears and might try to console the overly emotional participant. The therapists might also try to bring the participant back to the group by focusing on a specific task (reading or sharing an answer) or by trying to change the topic. At times, however, the participant's emotionality can become a burden on the group, constantly stalling discussions, forcing the attention back to him or her, and making it difficult for the group to meet the session's objectives.
  - Solution: The therapists need to make the participant feel heard with an empathic comment and perhaps a suggestion to discuss his or her issues during the socialization period, but they also need to move on and ensure that everyone benefits from the group.
- The wise: The wise participant is actually a great participant in many ways: He or she does all the exercises, quickly grasps concepts and techniques, and applies them to his or her daily life. We include this person with the "difficult" participants because he or

she is often a step ahead of everyone else and therefore tends to not participate much verbally and could become bored.

- Solution: The therapists should use this participant's input as much as possible, working with him or her to offer examples to the group or to assist others, somewhat as a peer co-therapist. If the wise participant is given a valued role, he or she will engage more in the group and participate in building stronger group cohesion, and everyone will benefit from his or her newly acquired understanding and application of CBT for psychosis concepts and techniques.

Conclusion

Various obstacles may arise when planning, setting up, or delivering group CBT for psychosis. Some of these obstacles are context-specific, whereas others are linked to clinicians or participants struggling in various ways when dealing with change. The examples given in this chapter are not exhaustive—other obstacles may present themselves in some settings, whereas particular participant types may be perceived as challenging by some therapists but not by others. We have had the opportunity to deliver workshops to experienced mental health clinicians and to train graduate students, in psychology and nursing, in delivering group therapy with various clienteles. We have at times been surprised to discover what or who is considered challenging for whom. For instance, many students will find the "overly emotional" participant extremely challenging, whereas more experienced therapists will have more trouble with the "delinquent" or "confronter." There are no magic answers regarding which intervention will be most useful when dealing with specific difficult participants. Similarly, co-therapy difficulties or challenges with management can be dealt with in various ways. We have offered suggestions stemming from our experience in running groups in various settings. There are certainly other ways to overcome these challenges and obstacles that could work as well, or perhaps even better.

Therapist Competence: What Skills Are Needed to Conduct Group CBT for Psychosis?

This chapter covers the typical clinician competencies such as empathy and warmth but also the necessary skills to conduct a group, such as time management, setting the agenda, using CBT techniques appropriately, and skillfully managing interactions in the group. This chapter will help clinicians better prepare themselves for running the group. We also describe existing measures for assessing therapist competence in CBT for psychosis, as well as in group CBT for psychosis.

What Is Competence?

Before attempting to describe or define competence, it is important to consider the relevance of therapist competence in the context of fairly structured approaches such as the group CBT for psychosis proposed in this book. A large body of research on the effects of psychotherapy methods and therapist competence suggests that who the therapist is makes a bigger difference than which method is used (Wampold, 2001). Although structured manuals help decrease outcome differences between therapists (Crits-Christoph et al., 1991), the best group CBT for psychosis workbook might be only as good as the therapists who will conduct the group. But what does it mean to be "good" or competent?

In the literature, there is no actual consensus regarding the definition of clinician competence, and the same is true for competence in group CBT for psychosis. In the psychotherapy literature, competence is often considered equivalent to experience: Those with many years of experience are de facto considered more competent than younger or less experienced therapists. This link appears intuitively sound: Someone who has conducted CBT with many individuals will likely be better at helping a wide range of individuals than someone who has recently learned CBT. Yet studies have shown that not all experienced therapists are competent, whereas some novice therapists can be quite competent, depending on the criteria used to determine competence (Brown et al., 2013). According to Ronnestad and Skovholt (2003), experience (i.e., number of years of practice) should not be confounded with therapist development, which implies improving oneself over time. Furthermore, experience can imply, for some, a certain degree of rigidity or resistance to trying new approaches or techniques. Given that group CBT for psychosis has been applied in certain clinics and settings for only about a decade, and that CBT for psychosis itself is not yet widely taught in academic settings, it would not make sense to consider experience or even therapist development as the only criterion for judging competence in group CBT for psychosis. It is, however, possible to determine a set of skills, abilities, and attitudes that a therapist should master in order to be considered a competent group CBT for psychosis therapist.

Competent Group CBT for Psychosis Therapists

As with all group therapies, group CBT for psychosis therapists need to constantly observe and address three levels:

- *The group level*: Keep in mind the theme being covered by the group today; make sure the group as a whole is doing well (no one is left out, good climate).
- *The interpersonal level:* Create parallels between participants, encourage interactions and interpersonal help, recognize and address conflicts.
- *The intrapersonal level*: Help each person work on his or her personal issues; make sure the group and themes are meeting each person's needs.

The group therapists do not need to constantly intervene on all three levels but should always be aware of what is going on at each level. Even when the group is following a workbook, various interactions are at play, and the group therapists need to stay alert in order to deal with the issues that might arise. The group and its participants might feel frustrated leaving the group if only one of the three levels was addressed during the entire session. This may be because the therapists spent all the time discussing individual issues for each person without linking these experiences to others, or they may have focused only on interactions or the day's theme without allowing time for personal disclosure. Competent group therapists will keep these three levels in mind and will try to make sure they are all addressed, even if briefly, during each session.

Other qualities and attitudes help define what we consider a good group CBT for psychosis therapist. The following is a list of general competencies that effective group therapists need to possess:

- *Warmth, understanding, and empathy:*

  As with most therapies, the group therapists need to express warmth, understanding, and empathy. These basic attitudes help create trust and facilitate the development of group cohesion. At times, a participant might be very confused, and it can be difficult for the therapists to understand what he or she is saying. The therapists do not have the luxury of spending 20 minutes with a single participant to verify their understanding and instead might have to express a more general form of empathy such as "It seems you are going through something very stressful at the moment."

- *Flexibility:*

  It might seem challenging to demonstrate flexibility while using a structured workbook with predetermined themes. Flexibility can mean finding ways of making links between a pressing issue that someone brings to the group and the theme planned for the session. For example, a participant in the group mentioned being very upset and was convinced he would be evicted from his apartment because his landlord mentioned he was going to conduct some renovations. This situation could be used for the group to practice concepts learned so far (such as checking the facts, seeking alternatives, rating his stress level, or trying new coping strategies), prior to tackling the day's theme. Or, depending on the day's planned session, the situation could also be used to illustrate the concept to be worked on, with the entire group trying, for instance, to seek facts (e.g., "Have you asked him if you needed to leave your apartment during the renovations?" "Did he say you needed to move?"). Flexible therapists are able to keep in mind their agenda while adapting to the situation at hand. At times, such as during an emergency (e.g., someone speaks of being suicidal), the planned agenda can be set aside with the group's approval.

- *Skill:*

  Here we use the term *skill* in the sense of using the CBT for psychosis skills or techniques well. This implies mastering the skill, for example, using Socratic questioning appropriately by carefully bringing the participant to realize that there are missing elements of proof supporting his or her distressful belief. Being skillful also implies being able to use different skills depending on the situation or the participant's current need. A participant might become very defensive, for instance, when trying to check the facts supporting his or her belief. A skillful therapist would quickly change strategies and might instead focus on trying to diminish the participant's distress by exploring coping strategies or the participant's strengths to deal with this belief. Therapists not only should be skillful in the application of one technique or concept but also should master multiple techniques and concepts and know when to use them, as well as when to encourage the group's participants to use them.

- *Timing:*

  The concept of timing includes both time management, which means that the session needs to be organized to provide enough time to complete the planned activities, and timing of an intervention, which is more about saying or doing the right thing at the right moment. For instance, therapists need to continually judge whether it is the right time to explore a sensitive topic or belief in more depth, whether they should let participants talk at greater length, or whether they should bring participants back on topic, given time constraints.

- *Creativity:*

  Creativity not only implies a degree of flexibility but also means thinking outside the box. What should the therapists do if all the participants who misused substances miss the session on substance misuse? Depending on the participants' preferences, reviewing a previous session that participants wish to discuss in more depth could be a solution, as could having a discussion on other addictive behaviors they might have (such as overeating, smoking cigarettes, gambling). How do therapists explain concepts that appear too abstract for some members in the group? They can use images or objects to illustrate their explanation. For instance, colored glasses might help some people realize that seeing things only in one color (or only in one way) is limiting. A half-full (or half-empty) glass of water can help explain the concept of pessimism. How do therapists get the participants to actively participate when everyone appears tired or withdrawn? Getting people to move around, stand on a chair, or sit on the floor can help them change their perspective and become more involved in the session. Asking people to change seats, to stretch, or to write on the flip chart can also lead to more participation in the session. Creative therapists will use the group members' input and might propose new ideas or activities when things do not go as planned. Creative therapists do not appear to get "stuck" in difficult situations, instead often finding original ways of making the group work optimally. It is not necessary to constantly be creative in each session, but it can be helpful to use creative solutions when problems arise.

- *Collaboration:*

  Competent group CBT for psychosis therapists do not run the sessions alone; they skillfully engage participants in collaboration with each other, helping other participants in various ways during the group sessions. As such, the participants do not spend the sessions talking to the therapists but instead interact among themselves, as well as with the therapists. The therapists model effective collaboration by working well together, in co-therapy, and by sharing explanations and activities, while also guiding participants in their interactions. For example, the therapists might instruct participants to address each other directly, or might always start by asking other participants to offer their answer to a question someone asked before answering it themselves.

Measuring Therapist Competence

Other than measuring years of experience, some studies have used scales to determine if therapists were competent in CBT for psychosis. These include the Cognitive Therapy Rating Scale (CTRS; Young and Beck, 1980), the Cognitive Therapy Scale—Revised (CTS-R; James, Blackburn, & Reichelt, 2001), and the Cognitive Therapy Scale for Psychosis (CTS-Psy; Haddock et al., 2001). All scales assess both general skills (such as agenda setting, interpersonal effectiveness) and specific skills (e.g., guided discovery, eliciting key behaviors or cognitions), with many overlapping domains in all three scales. The domains covered for each scale are presented in Table 13.1. The CTRS was the essential influence for the other two scales, which explains why they all use a similar 6-point anchoring system for each domain whereby a more competent therapist should obtain the highest scores.

The CTRS and the CTS-R have been used extensively in many studies. However, they both are fairly general CBT scales that do not take into consideration specificities linked to psychosis. The CTS-Psy, however, is psychosis-specific but seems skewed toward lower-level skills as most trained therapists obtain scores of 50% or lower (Haddock et al., 2001).

One of the problems with using these scales is that treatment fidelity and therapist competence are seen as interchangeable. Yet a therapist can apply CBT concepts and techniques "by the book" and obtain a high rating on these scales (demonstrating treatment fidelity) while at the same time being considered as fairly incompetent by his or her supervisor. These scales tap into CBT behaviors and attitudes, but the anchor points do not enable one to rate how appropriate the intervention was, if it really flowed, or if the client seemed to experience it as positive and helpful. These scales were also developed for CBT offered in individual therapy and do not offer cues regarding how to use the

TABLE 13.1 Domains covered in CTRS, CTS-R, and CTS-Psy

Domain Type	CTRS	CTS-R	CTS-Psy
General	Agenda	Agenda	Agenda
	Feedback	Feedback	Feedback
	Understanding	Interpersonal effectiveness	Understanding
	Interpersonal effectiveness	Collaboration	Interpersonal effectiveness
	Collaboration	Pacing and efficient use of time	Collaboration
	Pacing and efficient use of time		
Specific	Guided discovery	Guided discovery	Guided discovery
	Focusing on key cognitions and behaviors	Eliciting of appropriate emotional expression	Focusing on key cognitions
	Strategy for change	Eliciting key cognitions	Choice of intervention
	Application of CBT techniques	Eliciting and planning behaviors	Homework
	Homework	Conceptual integration	Quality of intervention
		Application of change methods	
		Homework	

anchor points for group CBT. Interpersonal effectiveness is different when dealing with one client versus a group of participants. Similarly, setting the agenda is quite different when using a structured workbook in a group than when choosing the session topics with an individual client.

Nonetheless, the elements mentioned in the CTRS and its various adaptations can also apply to group CBT for psychosis. In Table 13.2, we have attempted to use the CTRS domains to illustrate what a high competence score would be for a group CBT for psychosis therapist for each domain. Two domains were added: positive focus and cultural sensitivity. In previous chapters, we have discussed at length the importance of keeping a

TABLE 13.2 CTRS domains applied to group CBT for psychosis

Domains	Competence in Group CBT for psychosis (i.e., a high rating)
Agenda	Agenda is clearly set by including relevant review and describing today's theme, and asking the participants if they see the importance of the theme. If problems arise during the therapy (e.g., emotional breakdown, voices or paranoid thoughts flare up, conflicts between participants, therapist is confronted—accused of incompetence), the therapist sets the agenda aside and with tact and flexibility deals with the situation at hand.
Feedback	Appropriate feedback is asked or given frequently and at the right moments. If a participant does not offer the expected answer, the therapist makes a positive comment regarding the answer and tries a different strategy or a different angle that takes into account the participant's difficulty in understanding the concept (e.g., use of an image instead of words). The therapist is open to incorporating participants' suggestions and inputs. The therapist checks for understanding (i.e., the participants understand what he is saying), for agreement (i.e., the participants agree with the idea), or checks for the therapist's own understanding (i.e., to make sure that he or she is truly grasping what the participant is trying to say) with empathy and tact. The therapist creates a context where feedback happens naturally, where participants in the group and co-therapists "understand each other" by asking questions and using various creative tools to help (metaphors, graphs, drawings, cultural references, etc.).
Interpersonal effectiveness	The therapist appears genuinely interested in each participant, maintains eye contact, and is warm and authentic throughout the session. The therapist supports and offers positive regard (i.e., expresses genuine delight in successes and interest in participant) to each, not favoring one over others in the group, and is able to work through difficult situations such as breaks in the group cohesion (naming the situation, problem-solving). He or she is able to calm an agitated participant without becoming defensive or righteous, or to use himself appropriately and when needed (e.g., display true empathy and genuine caring). The therapist always interacts with participants in a warm and respectful way.
Collaboration	Excellent collaboration, with shared work (the group brings ideas and ways of initiating change to the table) throughout the session. When problems arise (e.g., a participant is clearly overwhelmed by his voices, is having difficulties that make him less trusting, or brings content that is clearly off topic), the therapist intervenes with skill, finding a way to collaborate on a common theme nonetheless. The therapist can use creative ways to involve the participants (e.g., asking people to work in pairs or asking a participant to write on the board).
Effective time use	Excellent use of time, with a clear beginning, middle, and end phase of the session. The time respect is flexible and creative, and the therapist knows when a digression is actually an important topic that needs addressing. Even when difficult topics arise (e.g., suicidal ideas or criticism), the therapist addresses the topic with tact and professionalism, while finishing on time and planning what is needed in the situation. Even with difficult situations, there is good flow—the therapist has a sense of time and knows how to effectively use it.

(continued)

TABLE 13.2 Continued

Domains	Competence in Group CBT for psychosis (i.e., a high rating)
Positive focus	The therapist uses a goal-oriented approach and skillfully uses positive concepts in various ways (homework, exercises, etc.), including concepts of self-esteem and self-compassion when appropriate. The therapist focuses on developing new strengths within each participant, as well as on creating strong group cohesion (through support, common values).
Accessing key emotions	The therapist addresses past and current emotions from more than one angle, helping participants recognize, self-attribute, recognize in others, and use self-regulation strategies or link emotions with key cognitions. Therapist uses himself as well as other participants' emotional reactions as examples.
Eliciting key cognitions	The therapist addresses current beliefs and thoughts during the session, helping participants recognize links with current and past emotions, behaviors, and situations, using the workbook and previously presented concepts to elicit thoughts. The therapist effectively uses him- or herself and the other participants in the group to help identify thoughts or beliefs. Participants' key cognitions are appropriately addressed and put in context during the group (e.g., emphasized to show their importance, or normalized).
Eliciting key behaviors	The therapist addresses current behaviors, trying to help participants recognize links with current and past emotions, thoughts, and situations, using the workbook and previously presented concepts to elicit behaviors. The therapist effectively uses him- or herself and the other participants in the group to help identify the role of the behavior and its impact. Participants' key behaviors are appropriately addressed and put in context (e.g., emphasized to show their importance or normalized). Negative behaviors or behaviors that might jeopardize the therapy are adequately dealt with during the session (or outside the group by the co-therapist).
Guided discovery	The therapist expresses curiosity regarding participants' beliefs, helps exploration without judgment or becoming collusive. Questioning by the therapist and the other participants allows participants to reflect upon their experiences, bringing them to consider other options. The therapist is highly effective in face of difficulties (e.g., a participant is defensive in response to questioning, participants in a group offer suggestions that are not helpful).
Conceptual integration	The vulnerability-stress-competence model and the A-B-Cs of CBT model are made clear and personalized, are explained in participants' own words, are linked to each new concept or technique learned or homework, and are referred to in the context of each person's goals.
Application of change methods (use of CBT for psychosis techniques)	The CBT for psychosis techniques used are well explained (using different means) to participants, repeated in appropriate context, well integrated by them during the session, are strengths based, and can easily be used by participants at home.
Cultural sensitivity	The therapist exhibits comfort, ease, and curiosity when discussing cultural issues. The therapist is willing to learn more about a specific topic and creatively incorporates culturally relevant information into interventions. May utilize appropriate self-disclosure to encourage process or may show insight and awareness if making cultural assumptions and work skillfully to repair this.
Homework	The therapist reviews the homework at the beginning of the session (with each participant) and explains the homework to the group and encourages participants to do the homework at the end of the session. Although the homework is predetermined and derived from the content of the session, the therapist helps participants personalize the homework, anticipate obstacles, and identify solutions.

positive focus in the group sessions. As for cultural sensitivity, it suggests that therapists are able to adapt to the cultural reality of the participants (e.g., linked to ethnic, religious, or age group references).

When Is Someone "Good Enough" to Conduct Group CBT for Psychosis?

Clinicians reading this chapter might feel uncertain regarding their competence, realizing that group therapy, particularly group CBT for psychosis, seems quite complex and involves multiple skills and abilities. Yet, as mentioned previously, participants do not expect therapists to be perfect or to always have the right answer or to propose the right intervention at exactly the right moment. There is room for error and room for improvement for the therapists who are "good enough" and who have insight into their actual performance during a group session.

By "good enough," we mean someone who is well prepared before a session. The therapist will take time to review the content of the session and go over the suggestions in this book pertaining to the session being prepared. The therapist will also make sure that the concepts and techniques that he or she will be presenting to the group are clear in his or her mind. The therapist will also anticipate how the session will go—trying to imagine how the group will interact during the session and preparing a "backup plan" or extra explanations if things do not go as intended. A good enough therapist also takes a few minutes to discuss with the co-therapist how they both foresee the session and how their roles should be shared. Essentially, a good enough therapist is first and foremost well prepared, enthusiastic, naturally warm, empathic, and understanding and confident in the usefulness of the group intervention offered.

A good enough therapist is also someone who is able to self-reflect that is, who is able to realize when things did not flow as they should have, or is able to see when a mistake was made or if a discussion got out of hand. A highly competent therapist might be able to quickly fix such problems as they arise, whereas the good enough therapist should be able to at least acknowledge them. Furthermore, he or she should try to find solutions in order to resolve the problem during the following session or to avoid having such situations repeated. Reviewing the competencies listed here, consulting with the co-therapist or with other colleagues, or seeking external supervision can also help the good enough therapist in his or her development toward competence. As with most skills, therapists need to "live and learn" by conducting more than one group CBT for psychosis to allow themselves to improve in their group and CBT for psychosis skills. The good enough therapist is essentially someone who has sufficiently mastered the skills we can think of as the three "knows":

1. *Know:* Basic knowledge in CBT for psychosis. The therapist knows the concepts and techniques that will be presented in the group and understands why they are useful and why they are presented in the order proposed.

2. *Know-how:* Understanding of group processes. The therapist recognizes the importance of the therapeutic factors in group CBT for psychosis and facilitates their development (by offering structure, clear goals, hope, cohesion, etc.). The therapist also knows how to present the CBT for psychosis concepts and techniques while facilitating these processes.

3. *Know-how-to-be:* Appropriate role and attitudes. The therapist displays the basic therapeutic attitudes (warmth, respect, empathy, etc.) and works well with the co-therapist to facilitate group learning and sharing. The therapist is authentic (recognizes own limits but seeks solutions) and finds a good balance between running the group and letting the participants run the group, while ensuring that the theme of the day is well covered and the session ends on time.

On the one hand, a good group therapist who masters well the "know-how-to-be" might have to improve his or her basic CBT for psychosis knowledge in order to master the CBT for psychosis techniques and concepts and apply them skillfully in the group. On the other hand, a highly skilled CBT for psychosis therapist might need to develop "know-how" and "know-how-to-be" skills that are more specific to group work. Therapists need to recognize their strengths and find ways to maximize them, and also recognize their limits and learn how to overcome them, to become competent group CBT for psychosis therapists.

Conclusion

This chapter has aimed at better defining competence in CBT for psychosis as well as in group therapy and more specifically in group CBT for psychosis. The domains listed here are not exhaustive but offer some guidelines to what we consider are some of the elements that make a competent group therapist. Many of these elements can be found in novice therapists (e.g., warmth, empathy, interpersonal effectiveness), whereas others might necessitate more time and experience to truly master (e.g., appropriate use and timing of techniques, intervening on all three levels: group, interpersonal, and intrapersonal). We also wished to detail how some competencies are reflected in specific domains of group CBT for psychosis, while ensuring that novice therapists who possess "good enough" skills feel encouraged to conduct group CBT for psychosis.

CBT Groups for Psychosis With Other Targets

Groups using CBT principles or techniques but targeting either a specific symptom or a domain outside of typical CBT for psychosis have been developed and tested. Some of these groups have been presented briefly in Chapter 3 and have demonstrated their empirical efficacy. In this chapter, we describe them in more detail. We present groups that focus on voices, self-esteem, stress management, and CBT for work integration and have also added a CBT group for parents or family members of individuals with psychosis, which seems to be effective.

Group for Voices

Til Wykes's group for voices is one of the first developed for individuals with psychosis that clearly uses CBT principles and techniques. As mentioned in Chapter 1, prior to the group for voices, few group interventions attempted to change individuals' perceptions of their symptoms or of themselves. A group therapy focused on voices seemed necessary for many reasons. Apart from cognitive deficits, hearing voices is one of the earliest signs of psychosis and one of the most distressing experiences for people with psychosis. There is also evidence that, for many (more than 30%), voices persist even after they have taken the prescribed levels of medication (Pantelis & Barnes, 1996). Furthermore, the experience of hearing voices often makes people feel alienated from others, whereas the group allows participants to realize they are not alone, somewhat normalizing their unusual experiences.

Group CBT for voices is offered over the course of seven sessions and uses a structured manual. The sessions' themes and content are presented in Table 14.1.

The group for voices has been validated in at least three randomized controlled trials. The initial wait-list-controlled study found significant improvements in the belief about the voices (e.g., their malevolence) and in self-esteem (Wykes, Reeder, Corner, Williams, &

TABLE 14.1 Group CBT for voices session content

Session Number and Theme	Session Content
1. Engagement and sharing of information about the voices	• Watch video about voices. • Discussion and normalization of voice experiences.
2. Exploring models of psychosis	• Watch video discussion of models of voices. • Compare psychological and medical models. • Discussion on psychological and medical treatments for voices. • Discussion on epidemiology of hearing voices.
3. Exploring beliefs about hallucinations	• Voices internal or external? • Explore power of voices (omnipotent, malevolent …). • Consequences if don't obey voices. • Verify if attempts to check facts linked to belief of voices.
4. Developing effective coping strategies	• Explore existing coping strategies and their effectiveness. • Present other coping strategies, which ones they might use and when? • Try a new coping strategy (homework).
5. Developing an overall model of coping with voices	• Review new coping strategies' effectiveness. • Discussion on stigma and labeling (beliefs linked with voices). • Discussion on medication and recreational drugs. • Try another new coping strategy (homework).
6. How to improve self-esteem	• Review of coping strategies' effectiveness. • Self-esteem game (write qualities on card). • Importance of positive self-regard and self-efficacy.
7. Follow-up session (2–6 weeks later)	• Review of coping strategies' effectiveness. • Presentation of the vulnerability-stress-competence model. • Review of the module (what was learned, liked, etc.).

Everitt, 1999), whereas the following trial found improvements in social behavior and also found greater improvements in severity of voices for those who received the group treatment with more experienced therapists (Wykes et al., 2005). A trial conducted in the United States by David Penn and colleagues (2009) used the same module but compared the effects to another intervention (supportive therapy) and found that the CBT group had significantly lower total and general symptoms, a near significant decrease in positive symptoms, and nonsignificantly higher levels of insight but showed no change in voice distress or intensity. A similar group has also been used with adolescents suffering from psychosis (Newton et al., 2005; Newton, Larkin, Melhuish, & Wykes, 2007), which showed that it was acceptable and achieved some change but that maintenance of the effects was affected by external events and influences (e.g., the family).

Self-Esteem Group: *I Am Super!*

Although many definitions of self-esteem exist, most describe it as a self-concept that can fluctuate with social feedback and self-evaluations (Bednar & Peterson, 1995; Crocker & Wolfe, 2001). As such, self-esteem develops—and is at times kept stable—through the critical evaluation an individual has of his or her reaction to difficult or stressful life events, which is then internalized as a personal characteristic, as well as from external feedback

(Bednar & Peterson, 1995). Understandably, environmental factors, such as stigma (Link, Struening, Neese-Todd, Asmussen, & Phelan, 2001; Thesen, 2001; Wright, Gronfein, & Owens, 2000), institutionalization (Estroff, 1989), and negative family interactions (Barrowclough et al., 2003) have been found to be detrimental to self-esteem in individuals with severe mental illness. Furthermore, studies have found links between self-esteem and social functioning (Bradshaw & Brekke, 1999; Brekke, Levin, Wolkon, Sobel, & Slade, 1993; Roe, 2003), perceived quality of life (Eklund, Backstrom, & Hansson, 2003; Sörgaard et al., 2002; Torrey, Mueser, McHugo, & Drake, 2000; Van Dongen, 1998), depression (Shahar & Davidson, 2003), and psychotic symptoms (Barrowclough et al., 2003; Shahar & Davidson, 2003; Sörgaard et al., 2002). Moreover, theorists and experimental psychologists have suggested links between low self-esteem and the development of paranoid delusions (Bentall, Corcoran, Howard, Blackwood, & Kinderman, 2001), as well as the maintenance of psychotic symptoms (Garety, Kuipers, Fowler, Freeman, & Bebbington, 2001).

For individuals with psychosis or another severe mental illness who present with low self-esteem and appear to lack motivation to actively participate in their recovery, the self-esteem group *I Am Super!* can be a useful tool. This structured group, empirically validated by Lecomte et al. (1999) in Canada and by Borras et al. (2009) in Switzerland, aims at increasing self-esteem in individuals suffering from psychosis. It is an adaptation of Reasoner's "Building Self-Esteem" module (Reasoner, 1992), originally conceived for children and adolescents in school contexts. It is one of the few existing structured group modules developed for the purpose of increasing self-esteem in individuals with schizophrenia.

The *I Am Super!* module is divided into five key building blocks: a sense of security, a sense of identity, a sense of belonging, a sense of purpose, and a sense of competence (see Table 14.2 for the list of activities covered):

- A sense of security implies feeling safe in one's environment, being able to trust others, relying on past experience to predict or anticipate events, and being aware of the environment's rules and regulations.
- A sense of identity refers to self-perception, which includes knowledge of one's strengths, weaknesses, and desires, and awareness of how one appears to others.
- A sense of belonging stems from feeling socially accepted and being part of a group that shares certain attributes.
- A sense of purpose includes the ability to reach self-determined goals, overcome obstacles, and take appropriate risks.
- A sense of competence is obtained by meeting challenges to achieve goals and experience success. One's sense of competence depends not only on possessing specific skills but also on believing that one can use them effectively and that one is worthy of happiness and fulfillment (Reasoner, 1992).

Although the I am Super module was inspired by a developmental approach, we consider it to be based on CBT principles because it aims at modifying dysfunctional

TABLE 14.2 Activities included in the *I Am Super!* module

Domain	Name of Session	Goal of Session
Sense of security	S-1: Where I live?	Make the living environment more secure and enjoyable.
	S-2: Responsibilities	Understand the value of being responsible.
	S-3: Trust	Realize the importance of trust and the difficulties in gaining it back once it is lost.
	S-4: Criticisms	How to deal effectively and positively with criticisms.
	S-5: What worries me	Share strategies to overcome fears and worries.
Sense of identity	I-1: Who am I?	Find positive statements to describe ourselves.
	I-2: Words that describe me	Recognize positive qualities in ourselves and in others in the group.
	I-3: Happiness	Explore what makes each person happy or feel better.
	I-4: My qualities	Realize positive qualities in various contexts, as well as what to improve.
Sense of belonging	A-1: Helping others	Acknowledge the value of helping others.
	A-2: Working with a partner	Learn the value of working with others, and practicing it.
	A-3: Affection	Realize the importance of showing affection and appreciation to someone special (and doing it).
	A-4: What I value	Recognize personal values shared with others.
Sense of purpose	P-1: Goals of the week	Break down long-term goals into smaller weekly goals.
	P-2: Changing negatives into positives	Find new ways of seeing negative situations.
	P-3: Thinking positively about myself	Determine how we would like others to perceive us.
	P-4: Personal development	Recognize personal strengths and aspects to improve (and how).
	P-5: Taking risks	Name challenges, rate the level of difficulty, and work to overcome one.
Sense of competence	C-1: I write myself a letter	Recognize strengths, accomplishments, and goals to meet.
	C-2: What I do well	Realize the contexts that enable us to achieve goals (alone, with others, with noise, etc.).
	C-3: Statements	Describe positive statements regarding ourselves as important, able, talented, nice, and worthy of respect.
	C-4: Strengths and weaknesses	Name strengths, accomplishments, and weaknesses that need working on.
	C-5: I rate myself	Identify living domains where one is autonomous or dependent on others (to work on the latter).
	C-6: Review	Review of the module (what was learned, liked, disliked, needs to continue working on, etc.).

beliefs about oneself and uses cognitive and behavioral strategies to help participants develop a healthier self-esteem. The group is cognitively simple, meaning that individuals who have important cognitive deficits but have basic reading and writing skills can benefit from it. It also involves homework, namely, applying the skills outside of the group, and setting and assessing goals for each week. We recommend that the group be offered twice a week for 3 months, although some have used it successfully once a week for 6 months. The *I Am Super!* module was validated through two large-scale studies. The first study, a randomized controlled trial, took place in Canada with individuals diagnosed with schizophrenia receiving long-term inpatient care (the average length of hospitalization was 14 years), with the group obtaining significant improvements in symptoms and in coping skills compared with the control group, which received treatment as usual (Lecomte et al., 1999). The second study was also a randomized-controlled trial, conducted in Switzerland and involving individuals receiving services in the community with or without rehabilitation and case management. This latter study found that the group was effective in improving self-esteem, self-assertiveness, symptoms, and active coping strategies, even more so for those receiving rehabilitation and case management (Borras et al., 2009). Both studies showed that it is possible to improve the self-esteem of people with psychosis or schizophrenia with the *I Am Super!* group module but that improvements can only be maintained when the environment is also involved, given the importance of feedback from others in maintaining a healthy self-esteem. It is possible to obtain a copy of the module at the following website: http://lespoir.ca.

A variant of the self-esteem module, focusing on self-esteem as well as on perceived stigma but over the course of only seven sessions, was also studied in a wait-list control design using repeated within-participant measures. The results suggested that even a brief self-esteem intervention can have beneficial clinical effects on the participants' self-esteem and symptoms, although a longer intervention might be needed for sustained effects on self-esteem (Knight, Wykes, & Hayward, 2006).

Stress-Management Group: Coping and Competence

The vulnerability-stress-competence model described by Anthony and Liberman (1986) opened the door to a multitude of psychosocial interventions aimed at improving protective factors that facilitate coping and competence in order to modulate the deleterious effects of psychobiological vulnerability and socioenvironmental stressors. Coping and competence were therefore considered protection against relapse and tools to facilitate recovery. Given the heightened vulnerability to stress experienced by most individuals with psychosis, and the plethora of stressors many describe experiencing daily, an intervention specifically targeting one's recognition of stressors and coping when faced with stress was warranted. Based on Lazarus and Folkman's (1984) model and Folkman's (1991) operationalization of coping, Leclerc and colleagues (2000) developed and validated the Coping and Competence stress management group module for people with schizophrenia. As with the self-esteem module, the Coping and Competence module consists of 24 sessions, delivered twice a week over the course of 3 months. The module involves seven domains, or steps, enabling participants to recognize symptoms of stress and develop specific coping skills (Table 14.3).

TABLE 14.3 The seven steps involved in the Coping and Competence module

Step	Goal	Description
1	Identifying stress	Checking list of items of symptoms of stress on mind, body, and emotions
2	Cognitive appraisal of stress	Identification of sources of stress; linking stress to symptoms of stress
3	Cognitive appraisal of change	Recognizing if stress is modifiable or not
4	Cognitive appraisal of resources	Problem-solving: listing solutions and resources and determining how useful they could be depending on the stressor
5	Selection of coping strategy	Choice of three solutions for dealing with each stressor; selection of preferred strategy
6	Use of selected coping strategy	Description of how the strategy or skill should be used; anticipate outcomes
7	Evaluation of the outcome	Assessment of the outcome (of having used the coping strategy); repeat from step 1 if outcome is less than desired

First, participants learn about the possible effects of stress on their body, mind (thoughts), and emotions through a list of possible symptoms of stress and are asked to identify those they have experienced previously. Second, notions about stress are discussed, and participants examine possible sources of stress in their daily activities: relationships, situations, places, special moments, thoughts, and physical condition. Participants then review which stressors are important for them and decide which ones they wish to discuss. With the help of the group, they learn to distinguish the changeable from the nonchangeable stressors in their lives. After a session on problem-solving and available resources, they are encouraged to list solutions that might help them deal with specific stressful situations. This entails classifying possible sources of information, emotional support, or tangible help needed to address such situations. Various solutions to stressful situations are discussed with the group to determine which solutions are preferred and will be used by whom. When possible, three solutions (active coping strategies) are considered for each changeable stressful situation.

When a situation is not changeable, possible coping strategies to deal with the stressor are discussed and practiced. Emotional regulation, avoidance, and changing one's perception of the situation (e.g., minimizing its importance), as well as relaxation techniques, are explored and tried for the stressors that have been discussed. For each of the coping strategies that are considered, participants share their expected outcome for using that strategy (and are asked to try it). When participants try a strategy outside of the group, they are asked to share the outcome and discuss the results with the group during the following session. All participants have an opportunity to go through this process many times during the 24 sessions.

The Coping and Competence module was empirically validated in a randomized controlled trial with individuals with schizophrenia who had been receiving psychiatric services for many years (Leclerc et al., 2000). The results showed that the group was effective in improving psychotic symptoms, self-esteem, and specific independent living skills. Although the group has been offered to individuals with a long psychiatric history and who also had important cognitive deficits, it is slightly more demanding intellectually than the self-esteem module and can also be delivered to individuals who function well socially but need extra help dealing with the stressors in their lives.

Group CBT for Supported Employment

Supported employment programs are highly effective in helping people with severe mental illness obtain competitive jobs quickly (Bond, Drake, & Becker, 2008). However, only about 50% of those receiving such services obtain employment, and for those who do, job tenure is often a problem for many (Corbière & Lecomte, 2009). Of the various obstacles to job tenure that have been documented, dysfunctional beliefs regarding the workplace and one's own abilities have been proposed as a therapeutic target. Lysaker and colleagues (Davis, Lysaker, Lancaster, Bryson, & Bell, 2005) developed a group CBT for vocational rehabilitation for veterans with severe mental illness to help them recognize and correct dysfunctional beliefs relevant to work (e.g., "I expect to fail," "Everyone will dislike me," and "I expect this will all go perfectly"). Given the positive results of their Indianapolis Vocational Intervention Program (IVIP) in terms of better job maintenance, work performance, and self-esteem than for those in the control condition receiving standard services (Lysaker, Bond, Davis, Bryson, & Bell, 2005), we chose to adapt and shorten the program so it could be administered within supported employment programs. The group module known as Cognitive-Behavior Therapy for Supported Employment (CBT-SE; Lecomte, Lysaker, & Corbière (2009) consists of eight sessions over the course of 1 month, to respect the rapid job search principle of supported employment programs. The content was tailored to facilitate exploring cognitions and skills specific to the workplace, such as recognizing and managing one's stressors at work, determining and modifying dysfunctional thoughts (e.g., not jumping to conclusions, finding alternatives, seeking facts), overcoming obstacles (e.g., problem-solving), improving one's self-esteem as a worker (recognizing strengths and qualities), dealing with criticism, using positive assertiveness, finding coping strategies (for symptoms and stress) to use at work, negotiating accommodations, and overcoming stigma. The breakdown of the module is presented in Table 14.4.

A trial is currently underway, with half the participants receiving both supported employment and CBT-SE (N = 80) and the other half receiving only supported employment (N = 80). The baseline data on all the participants were collected when this chapter was written but the 1-year follow-up data had not all been collected. Preliminary results have been published on the first 24 participants who have completed the 12-month follow-up, including 12 participants who received at least three sessions out of the eight group sessions, and 12 participants who received only supported employment (Lecomte, Corbière, & Lysaker, 2014). In terms of feasibility and acceptability, therapists and participants all mentioned appreciating the group and finding it useful and helpful; some even mentioned feeling grateful to have had the opportunity to receive the intervention. In terms of work outcomes, 50% of all participants in both conditions found competitive work. Among those working competitively, the number of participants working more than 24 hours per

TABLE 14.4 CBT-SE session titles and content

Session number	Title	Content
1	Coping with stress at work	Recognizing stress, its effects on body, thoughts, emotions
		Recognizing stress in the various steps of work integration (interview, first day, etc.)
		Sharing strategies to cope with stress at work
2–3	Recognizing and modifying my dysfunctional beliefs linked to work	Learning the ABC's of CBT
		Understanding the impact of negative or dysfunctional beliefs on our emotions and behaviors
		Getting facts and finding alternative beliefs
4	Overcoming obstacles linked to reintegrating the workplace	Recognizing personal obstacles to obtaining or maintaining a job
		Sharing and practicing strategies to overcome these obstacles
5	My strengths and competencies related to work	Understanding the power of negative self-attributions
		Recognizing one's strengths and abilities with the help of others in the group
6	Accepting criticism and asserting myself appropriately	Using techniques learned so far when confronted with criticism (coping with stress, A-B-C, check facts, not jump to conclusions, recognize strengths)
		Learn relaxation and acceptance
		Role-play polite self-assertion
		Negotiating work accommodation with employer
7–8	My best coping strategies for work	Discussing disclosure of mental illness and stigma at work
		Reviewing coping strategies that work best for each person for personal stressors, symptoms, moods, and thoughts at work
		Review of the manual, what was learned, liked, etc.

week at the 12-month follow-up was higher in the CBT-SE group than in the control condition (75% vs. 50%). Similarly, there was a trend toward the number of consecutive weeks worked at the same job being slightly superior at the 12-month follow-up for those who had received the CBT-SE intervention (22.5 weeks vs. 18.3 weeks). These results should be considered with caution given that only 24 participants were looked at, whereas the final sample size will be 160 participants. Nonetheless, these preliminary results are promising. Furthermore, additional information regarding the impact of the CBT-SE intervention on the capacity to overcome obstacles at work, on self-esteem as a worker, and on other work-related variables has been collected and will be analyzed with the final sample soon.

Group CBT for Families of Individuals With Psychosis: Wellness-Inform-Talk-Help

When we started our trial on group CBT for psychosis, we received several phone calls from parents of individuals with psychosis who were taking part in the group. Parents wanted to learn more about CBT for psychosis and were wondering if we could also offer them some support. We therefore developed a multiple-family group therapy based on our group CBT for psychosis module called Wellness, Inform, Talk, Help (WITH), which not only aims to offer an understanding of CBT for psychosis but also encourages parents to use CBT techniques for themselves, in their own lives. The module also covers expectations, recovery, and expressed emotion, as well as ways of helping family members recognize their own limits as caregivers. The WITH module can be offered over the course of 16 hours or up to 24 hours. In clinics where the parents accompany their loved ones for each group CBT for psychosis session (such as in regions with poor public transportation), the WITH module can be offered in parallel to group CBT for psychosis, for the same length of time and at the same frequency (i.e., 24 sessions, twice a week for 3 months). It can also be offered in a briefer version (16 hours), but with longer sessions (i.e., 2 hours instead of 1 hour per session). The WITH module was designed to be attended by parents, without the family member with psychosis. Other family therapies exist that aim at working with the entire family together. Our goal was to offer tools that could help parents become better caregivers while giving them the space to share with other parents the challenges encountered when living with someone with a psychotic disorder. The content essentially follows the four sections of the group CBT for psychosis module but with added information and discussions on recovery, expressed emotions, and the parent's role as a caregiver. As with the group CBT for psychosis module, the parents are asked to reflect on questions, share their answers, and at times practice skills or strategies at home. Table 14.5 illustrates each section and the themes that are discussed.

Given that the WITH module also aims at educating parents on CBT, it is considered more of a hybrid psychoeducation-CBT group approach rather than a true CBT group. We did, however, expect it would help parents, so we conducted a pilot study with 40 parents who participated in the 16-hour version of the WITH multiple-family group. Although significant changes in perceived support were not detected, the results showed a significant clinical and statistical decrease in psychological distress in the parents who took part in the group, compared with their baseline scores. The qualitative information obtained also suggests that the group was appreciated and that the parents had integrated some CBT skills, as well as notions regarding recovery and how to maintain a healthier relationship with their relative who is receiving psychiatric care. Most agreed that the WITH group had been helpful and that they had a better understanding of and a better relationship with their family member with psychosis (Leclerc & Lecomte, 2012). It would have been best to compare the WITH module with another multiple-family intervention to determine if it offers better results. We did, however, learn that the previous multiple-family group offered in the clinics participating in our study had a very high dropout rate (more than 80%), whereas we had a dropout rate of less than 20%. The WITH module is still offered in the clinics that participated in our study, as well as in community organizations that offer support to family members of people with schizophrenia. We believe it offers not only support and information but also actual tools that parents can use for themselves and with their family member with psychosis.

TABLE 14.5 WITH module sections and themes

Section	Themes
1. Stress: How it impacts my life	Goals of the WITH module
	First episode, stress, and recovery
	Stress and symptoms
	Sources of stress
	Expressed emotions
	Protective factors
2. Verify hypotheses and look for alternatives	Cognitive behavioral therapy:
	Beliefs and their impact on emotions and behaviors
	Normalization
	Alternatives and verification of facts
	Socratic questioning
	The downward spiral ...
3. Drugs, alcohol, and states of mind	Values and social adherence
	Positive approach and self-esteem
	Drugs and alcohol
	Depression and suicidal ideation
	Modifying your mood
	Mindfulness
4. Coping and competence	Reduce symptoms by coping
	Support the person in reaching goals
	Family and friends' expectations
	Knowing how to support a close family member
	Knowing how to be
	The distinction between the role of a CBT therapist and of family members
	Module review

Conclusion

This chapter has aimed at presenting other groups for individuals with psychosis that our team has developed and that are related to group CBT for psychosis. Some of these focus on symptoms, such as the group on voices, whereas others aim at improving different aspects of one's experience of psychosis, such as coping with stress or improving self-esteem. As we have tried to illustrate here, CBT can help people in many ways, such as in managing thoughts and behaviors at work or in being a better caregiver for a family member with psychosis. More studies are warranted for some of these group interventions; a group module becomes recognized as an effective intervention only when it has demonstrated positive and clinically significant results in more than one randomized controlled trial (and ideally not conducted in the same setting). Nonetheless, to date, the groups proposed here have all obtained positive and interesting results in trials, or they show promising results and are being studied in more depth.

Conclusion

The Future of Group CBT for Psychosis

Cognitive behavioral therapy for psychosis has now established itself as an evidence-based intervention. Group CBT for psychosis might grow in popularity for several reasons: (a) Many clinical settings have high clinician-client ratios, making it very difficult to offer individual CBT for psychosis to those who need it; (b) few settings have sufficiently trained individual CBT for psychosis therapists; (c) financial constraints encourage clinics to support manualized group interventions when possible; and (d) all the studies to date using the group CBT for psychosis described in this book have obtained positive and clinically significant results.

The group CBT for psychosis workbook presented in detail in this book is currently being used in many countries around the world. Other group CBT for psychosis workbooks exist. Ours, however, is one of the few that has carefully considered the importance of therapeutic factors (such as group cohesion), the timing for introducing the various CBT for psychosis techniques and strategies, and giving the group a positive focus. Brief interventions seldom allow enough time to truly develop group cohesion, whereas 24 sessions are more than enough. Groups that repeat concepts and include new participants at any given time are perhaps easier for a clinic to run, but they do not benefit from the effects of group cohesion and of incremental learning. Focusing only on symptoms can be experienced as 'heavy' or depressing for participants; having a positive focus and including self-esteem activities make the groups appealing and increase the effects of the therapy. As mentioned in this book, group CBT for psychosis is effective when the essential therapeutic factors are present and with "good enough" therapists, therefore allowing the exploration of new behaviors and new ways of thinking. Furthermore, group CBT for psychosis works in accordance with the current recovery model, putting the person's goals and needs at the center of the treatment and suggesting, rather than imposing, tools that participants will choose (or not choose) to use.

Cognitive behavioral therapy–inspired groups for people with psychosis have been developed and have obtained promising results. New integrative approaches using group CBT for psychosis strategies or principles are likely to emerge in years to come. Integrative psychotherapy approaches are fairly common for psychologists working with clients presenting with other types of disorders or issues but are fairly novel for people with psychosis (Lecomte & Lecomte, 2012). Modified group CBT for psychosis is being offered within supported employment programs, along with social skills training, and also in some settings within dual-disorder programs for people with substance misuse disorders. We anticipate that group CBT for psychosis could be adapted for specific comorbid issues (such as social anxiety) or to help with other aspects of recovery, such as in developing healthy romantic relationships.

Some CBT for psychosis groups have also integrated third wave strategies, namely, mindfulness activities, into their sessions. Despite the number of articles and claims to date, few rigorous empirical studies on mindfulness have been conducted. A recent meta-analysis on mindfulness interventions in psychosis (Khoury, Lecomte, Gaudiano, & Paquin, 2013) included mostly nonrandomized and noncontrolled studies, found no effects on positive symptoms and only some modest effects on negative symptoms, but the interventions seemed to have some effect on other symptoms (such as anxiety or depression). The quality of these studies was generally poor, and most of them involved individual mindfulness, with few investigating group interventions. Most group studies are small and uncontrolled, and no group differences were found (e.g., Ruddle, Mason, & Wykes, 2011). Feasibility group studies from our team using mindfulness, acceptance, and compassion found that participants appreciated the group sessions but had difficulties grasping metaphors; they appeared to improve in emotional self-regulation, anxiety, depression, and somatic concerns but not in psychotic symptoms (Khoury, Lecomte, Comtois, & Nicole, 2013). Future rigorous studies are warranted to determine if groups using these techniques are effective in helping people with psychosis (or people with psychosis and comorbid mood or anxiety disorders), and if they have an added value when integrated with group CBT for psychosis.

Some studies also suggest that young individuals with psychosis might benefit from "virtual" CBT for psychosis groups, that is, online group forums that guide participants in using CBT for psychosis and enable them to share experiences with other participants (Alvarez-Jimenez et al., 2013). These e-health approaches will grow in popularity but should not decrease the appeal for "live" group CBT for psychosis. Many individuals with psychosis feel isolated and seek real person-to-person contact, whereas forum or Internet exchanges are often considered more impersonal and provide little opportunity to test out real-life social exchanges.

Conclusion

We expect that group CBT for psychosis is here to stay for many years to come. Variants might be proposed, and new technologies developed, but the need for people to come together to share experiences and learn new and useful strategies to help them during their recovery will remain. As clinicians, if you decide to run the group CBT for psychosis proposed here and would like to share your experience with us, feel free to contact us via our website http//: lespoir.ca.

The Group CBT for Psychosis Workbook

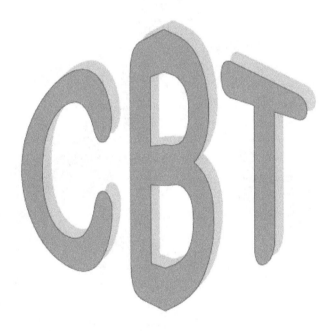

Cognitive-Behavioral Therapy

PARTICIPANT'S WORKBOOK

BY

Tania Lecomte, Ph.D.,

Claude Leclerc, Ph.D. &

Til Wykes, Ph.D.

2001

INTRODUCTION

The "CBT" module aims at understanding our symptoms better and finding new ways to deal with them and feel better about ourselves. The module consists of four parts, which are 1) *Stress: how it affects me*, 2) *Testing hypotheses and looking for alternatives*, 3) *Drugs, alcohol and how I feel*, and 4) *Coping and competence*.

Each part is described as we encounter it in the related activities. The CBT module follows the order of the activities in this workbook. Discussions are planned for each activity and are carried out, either in pairs or with the whole group discussing each topic. Following each activity, we will review what has been learned, what was liked or disliked and what was experienced. Each activity will end with a snack and socialization period.

STRESS: HOW IT AFFECTS ME

Learning objectives:

After having completed the activities in this section, each participant should be able to achieve the following objectives:

1. The participant is able to describe how stress can affect someone physically, mentally and emotionally.
2. The participant can describe in his/her own words the vulnerability-stress-competence model.

Activities:

S-1:	Introducing ourselves
S-2:	What is stress?
S-3:	What do I consider stressful?
S-4:	How I experience my symptoms
S-5:	Vulnerability-stress-competence model
S-6:	A personal goal

S-1: Introducing ourselves

Today's activity is meant to get to know each other better. Take a few minutes to answer each questwion before sharing your answer with the group.

1. Where do you live?

_____

_____

_____

_____

2. Who's your favorite musician or band?

_____

_____

_____

_____

3. What do you like to do, what are your interests?

_____

_____

_____

_____

4. Name a quality you have that others appreciate:

_____

_____

_____

_____

Once the discussion is over, we will review what we learned, what we want to remember, and what we liked or disliked.

5. What are you good at?

_____

_____

_____

_____

What I wish to remember:

_____

_____

_____

_____

S-2: What is stress?

Today's activity will help us understand what stress is and how it can change the way we feel and think. After discussing the possible effects of stress on your body, your mind and your emotions, we will share with the group the most common effects of stress in our daily lives.

A definition of stress:

Stress is a normal human reaction with effects on the body, the mind and the emotions. The first explanation of what is stress was given by Hans Selye, a researcher working in Montreal in the mid 20th century. He was interested by the reaction to stimulation: the experience of stress. He discovered how we react to danger: we can fight or we can run away 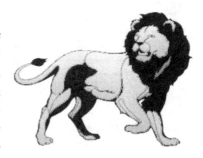 until we get exhausted. Either way a lot is happening to the body, the mind and the emotions. These reactions are the effects of stress and they arise when the person is experiencing an important event.

A. An important event:

People are not the same and they don't attribute the same importance to similar events. The same event can have a completely different meaning or importance for two different people. For example, losing 20 dollars can be very dramatic for one person and not at all important for another person.

1. Name an important event for you:

_____

_____   _____

_____

_____

B. The effects of stress can be experienced physically:

2. Look at these possible physical effects of stress and check (✓) the most frequent ones you have experienced:

☐ My heartbeat is faster
☐ I can't fall asleep
☐ I wake up often during the night
☐ I sleep too much, more than usual
☐ I feel tired
☐ I feel weak
☐ I sweat more than usual
☐ My voice trembles
☐ I feel sick (nausea) or I throw up
☐ I am not hungry
☐ I can't stop eating

☐ My cheeks turn red (blush)
☐ I turn pale
☐ My mouth is dry
☐ I feel aches all over my body
☐ My muscles become tense
☐ I constantly have to go to the bathroom
☐ I can't stop moving
☐ I can't stop doing the same thing over and over again
☐ I need to walk all the time
☐ I feel numb

☐ Other: (describe)_____

C. Effects of stress can be experienced in your mind:

3. Look at the list of possible effects of stress on the mind and check the most frequent ones you have experienced:

☐ My ideas are speeding up
☐ I feel like I am trapped
☐ I don't know what to think
☐ I have doubts about everything
☐ I can't remember anything
☐ I can't get rid of a thought
☐ My ideas are not clear
☐ I want to forget everything

☐ I am too excited and I can't clear up my mind
☐ I am thinking only about bad things
☐ I can't understand what is going on
☐ I can't get over a detail about the event and I am losing track of "the big picture"
☐ I can't concentrate
☐ I can't organize my thoughts

☐ Other: (describe)_____

D. Effects of stress can be experienced by different emotions:

4. Look at the list of possible effects of stress on emotions and check the most frequent ones you have experienced:

☐ I feel afraid
☐ I feel like hiding away, isolating myself from everyone
☐ I feel responsible for a situation that I didn't cause
☐ I feel discouraged
☐ I don't want to do anything
☐ I can't calm down
☐ I don't care about my physical appearance or hygiene
☐ I want everything to stop
☐ I want to do something crazy
☐ I am angry
☐ Other: (describe)_____

☐ I want to hurt someone
☐ I want to disappear
☐ I don't want to talk to anyone
☐ I don't recognize myself
☐ I feel like dirt
☐ I don't trust my best friends
☐ I feel guilty
☐ I don't trust myself
☐ I want to solve a problem by acting aggressively against someone or something
☐ I feel I am losing control of myself

_____

Homework: Fill out the "Effects of stress" sheet in the Annex this week

As a group, we will review what is an important event and try to identify the most common effects of stress in our lives.

What I wish to remember:

_____

_____

_____

_____

S-3: What do I consider stressful?

Stressful events happen all the time, but everyone reacts more or less intensely depending on the specific situation. Today we will focus on what is really stressful for each one of us.

Being evaluated or judged by people.

Getting into a fight with a parent.

Driving in heavy traffic.

Being hospitalized.

These are all examples of situations that might cause stress physically or psychologically. Think of five situations that might be stressful for you. These situations can be related to people, places, or events.

1. I feel stress when _____

_____

2. For me, it is stressful to _____

_____

3. I know I get stressed out if _____

_____

4. Though it doesn't happen often, this can cause stress for me:_____

_____

5. Not at first, but in the long run it becomes stressful for me to_____

_____

Circle one of the five examples you have mentioned and think of that stressor to evaluate your stress level, using the following page.

> **Once the discussion is finished, we will look back at why it's important to assess our stress level and to identify our stressors.**

MY STRESS LEVEL

Level 0	**Feeling good**
	I am calm, at peace with myself.
Level 1	**Minimal stress**
	I feel a little nervous, or agitated. It is temporary and I don't mind.
Level 2	**Light stress**
	I feel a little discomfort and I am trying to understand what is going on.
Level 3	**Moderate stress**
	Effects on my body, mind and emotions, but I am still in control. I can go on.
Level 4	**Important stress**
	I feel strange, uncomfortable. My heart is pounding and my muscles are tense. I am trying to find out how to stay in control.
Level 5	**Anxiety**
	I don't breathe easily, I'm feeling strange, or dizzy. I am afraid I am oing to lose control. I want to run away.
Level 6	**Moderate anxiety**
	My heart is pounding, I feel disoriented, like if it was not real. I can't breathe normally. I can't control myself any longer.
Level 7	**Panic**
	It is physically painful. I am afraid, I think I'm going to lose my mind. I am afraid of dying, I want to run away and escape right now.

What I wish to remember:

_____

_____

_____

_____

Homework: Fill out the "Stress Level" sheet in the Annex this week.

S-4: How I experience my symptoms

When we take the time to better understand ourselves, it becomes easier to deal with stress and find ways to feel better. Together we will discuss the following questions.

Think of the first time you were hospitalized in psychiatry or that you consulted someone concerning disturbing thoughts or symptoms. Try to recall how you felt at the time and how things have changed for you.

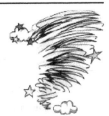

1. Why did you get help or why do you think you were hospitalized?

_____

_____

_____

_____

2. What did you think, see or hear?

_____

_____

_____

_____

Do you still think, see or hear the same things now?

_____

_____

_____

_____

3. How did you feel when you first got help?

_____

_____

_____

_____

Do you still feel the same way?

_____

_____

_____

_____

4. What's your understanding of what has been going on in your life for the past year or two ... how do you explain it?

_____

_____

_____

_____

We will review what was said, what you wish to remember and why it's important to make sense of our experiences.

What I wish to remember:

_____

_____

_____

_____

S-5: Vulnerability-stress-competence model

Now that we know more about stress, we will discuss a model explaining how stress can challenge our health. We will also look at how to prevent the negative effects of stress in our life.

Important things to know and remember:

The knowledge about stress has evolved a lot since Selye's work in the 1940's. Many questions arose and some got answered. For instance, it is now proven that the same stressful event does NOT cause the same stressful reactions in each person.

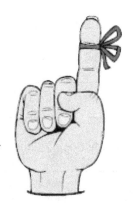

The explanation for this is that each one of us has a different vulnerability to some illness or reaction. Stress, especially a lot of stress, will favor the development of one or more of these reactions or illnesses.

How can we be vulnerable to a particular reaction or illness?

Our heredity and some events or accidents in our past may have caused that vulnerability. Some will be vulnerable to cholesterol or diabetes, some others will gain weight more easily than others while some might be vulnerable to mental health problems. "The Vulnerability-Stress-Competence Model," developed by Anthony and Liberman demonstrates this phenomenon.

"The Vulnerability-Stress-Competence Model" describes one's vulnerability as biological and psychological, causing specific challenges one has to deal with. This model also identifies how stress can amplify a health problem like psychotic symptoms, and how it is possible to protect ourselves by developing protective factors. The strength of these protective factors will affect the way we recover from an illness or stressful reaction.

1. *What do you think are your protective factors?*

_____

_____

_____

_____

2. *Here's a list of protective factors suggested by the model, personalize it by filling it in with one or more words for each factor.*

Protective Factors:
• Medication

_____

_____

• My Social Skills and Competence:

_____

_____

• My Coping Skills, Stress-Management and Self-Esteem:

_____

_____

• My Family and Social Support:

_____

_____

Definitions:
• *medication*: *drugs prescribed by your doctor or psychiatrist ... if you take them, what are they? Do you know what they are useful for?*
• *social skills and competence*: *abilities to talk to people, to ask for information or help when needed and to make friends.*
• *coping skills, stress-management and self-esteem*: *things you think about, say or do to feel better about yourself or to control your stress level or to diminish your symptoms (we will cover many in this group).*
• *family and social support*: *everyone who can offer support to you, counting family, friends, mental health staff, or others.*

My negative outcomes without protective factors

Name 4 problems you are facing in relation to your vulnerability:

1. _____

   _____

2. _____

   _____

3. _____

   _____

4. _____

   _____

Definition: *negative outcomes consist of all of the difficulties you have encountered in regards to your vulnerability such as symptoms, problems concentrating, not wanting to see people as much, etc.*

> *Let's look at "The Vulnerability-Stress-Competence Model" on the next page and see how it all fits together.*

VULNERABILITY STRESS COMPETENCE MODEL

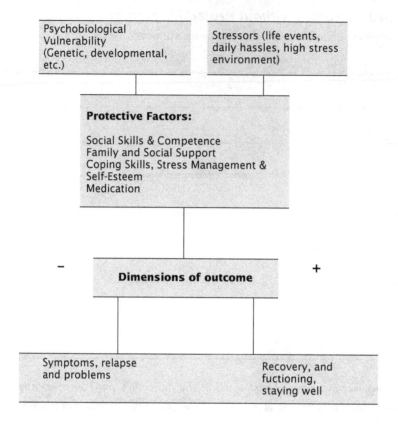

It's important to remember that COPING consists of all of the different ways we have to deal with or manage a problem, a challenge, or a difficult situation. Healthy SELF-ESTEEM means that one feels capable of managing life's challenges and feels worthy of happiness.

> **We will review what was said about "The Vulnerability-Stress-Competence Model." We will try to find out how this model could help us to understand what is going on during situations that might create stress.**

What I wish to remember:

_____

_____

_____

_____

S-6: A personal goal

It is important to be able to set goals and reach them in order to find a sense of purpose in our lives. Every day of the week can offer the opportunity to accomplish something, or to meet a small personal goal.

Make a list of things you would like to work on. For instance, you can think of how to stay well or how to diminish the impact stress has on you.

List:

_____

_____

_____

_____

_____

_____

_____

_____

_____

_____

For every day of the week, or for certain days, write a realistic goal from your list that you would like to meet.

At the end of the day, or the next morning, rate yourself in regards to having met your goal or not. It is best to think of small goals that are easily reached. When you meet your goal, make sure to tell the others in your group.

This goal sheet is yours, you are the judge of your own progress. You have many more of these sheets in the Appendix.

Day	Goal	Not met	Partly met	Met
Monday				
Tuesday				
Wednesday				
Thursday				
Friday				
Saturday				
Sunday				

Homework: Score this "Goal of the week" sheet at the end of everyday, starting today.

What we learned and remember about stress: How it affects me:

1. _____

_____

_____

2. _____

_____

_____

3. _____

_____

_____

4. _____

_____

_____

5. _____

_____

_____

Testing hypotheses and looking for alternatives

Learning objectives:

After having completed the activities in this section, each participant should be able to achieve the following objectives:

1. The participant is able to describe the ABC's of CBT, i.e. that the way we think about an event will influence the way we feel, act and react.
2. The participant is able to identify at least two hypotheses explaining different situations.
3. The participant is able to document facts to support his/her beliefs or can consider other alternatives.

Activities:

T-1: The ABC's of CBT

T-2: Common experiences

T-3: The traffic jam

T-4: How not-to-jump-to conclusions

T-5: Considering alternatives for my own beliefs

T-6: Looking at things from a positive perspective

T-1: The ABC's of CBT

Our behaviors and our emotional reactions to events are strongly affected by how we think about the events. Our thoughts are also influenced by many things such as our past, our perception and our own view of ourselves.

Watch the movie excerpt ... What do you think is going on? (If you've seen it before, what does the person who's watching think is going on?)

_____

_____

_____

_____

_____

For each example listed, try to imagine yourself in that situation and describe what you would think and how you would feel and act.

A for Antecedent What's the situation	B for Belief What do I think is going on?	C for Consequence 1) How do I feel? 2) What do I want to do?
1. Two of my friends stop talking as soon as they see me		1) 2)
2. My new girl friend (or boy friend) seemed angry and canceled our date		1) 2)
3. The bus driver is looking at me funny		1) 2)
4. Find your own example. . .		1) 2)

> *As a group, we will discuss the importance of verifying our thoughts and confirming our perceptions with facts.*

What I wish to remember:

_____

_____

_____

_____

T-2: Common experiences

Today we will discuss strange or difficult experiences we might have had lately and see how many of us have experienced similar things.

In the 1970's, researchers conducted experiments where people would be put in a "sensory deprivation" capsule where they could not hear, see or feel anything. Can you guess what people experienced after as little as 40 minutes?

80% reported hearing voices and seeing things that were not there...

Similar experiences happen for instance to people in mourning and to people having gone without sleep for many hours.

1. Do you ever hear voices or see things that no one else could hear or see?

   If yes, can you describe when it happens, what type of voice or image it is, what it says and how it makes you feel to experience that ?

   _____

   _____

   _____

   _____

Sometimes, either because they're tired or because they've had a bad experience in the past, people think others are out to get them, that someone might wish them harm. Others can think they hold specific powers or that they were chosen for a specific purpose, but no one seems to believe them.

2. Do you ever think people are out to get you or that you have powers or that you were chosen for a mission, but no one believes you?

   If yes, can you describe when it happens, who is out to get you, what type of powers you have or what's the mission you were chosen for?

   _____

   _____

   _____

   _____

3. Describe the impact these experiences (seeing or hearing things) or thoughts have on your behavior. What do you do or what do you refrain yourself from doing because of them?

_____

_____

_____

_____

What I wish to remember:

_____

_____

_____

_____

Homework: Fill out a new "Goal of the week" sheet in the Annex, using concepts we have seen so far.

T-3: The traffic jam

As a group, we will apply the axiom: "Any event can have several alternative explanations depending on the observer."

Try to find at least two answers for each question.

1a What causes a traffic jam?

_____

_____

_____

1b How can you know for sure?

_____

_____

_____

2a What might explain a scene where two people force a pedestrian into a car?

_____

_____

_____

2b How can you find out the real reason?

_____

_____

_____

3a What might explain that people are staring at you?

_____

_____

_____

3b How can you find out?

_____

_____

_____

> *Together, we will review why it's important to consider different alternatives before making an interpretation.*

What I wish to remember:

_____

_____

_____

_____

T-4: How not-to-jump to conclusions

We often make interpretations or decisions based on very little facts. Yet, we have learned so far how it is easy to misinterpret an event or situation. Today, we will explore how to prove or disprove our hypotheses before jumping to conclusions.

Checking information before believing a story is like the job of a detective. Each source must be investigated and every aspect of the story verified. For each example, explain how you would investigate the facts. You can use the cues to help you out.

Detective cues:

Who did it happen to?

Where did it happen?

Was anyone else involved?

Any witnesses?

Has any such thing ever happened before?

Why did it happen to that person?

Are there any other possible explanations for the event?

Andrew, a man recently laid-off from work, calls the police saying that aliens abducted him. He claims they put a probe in his head that allows them to hear his thoughts and control him. They also speak to him through this probe.

1. What facts do we need to check out the story?

_____

_____

_____

Sophie tells you she has special powers that allow her to predict the future.

She asks you to keep it secret because the government is paying people to follow her everywhere and watch her, even her family is being paid.

2. What facts do we need to check out the story?

_____

_____

_____

What I wish to remember:

_____

_____

_____

_____

Homework: Think of a thought that caused stress and fill out the "ABC's of CBT" sheet in the Annex.

T-5: Considering alternatives for my own beliefs

We have seen how our thoughts and perceptions of events can influence our emotions and behaviors. We have seen that these thoughts can be biased, and that we should consider alternatives and gather facts before jumping to conclusions. Now let's see if we can do these exercises with our own beliefs.

At times, because of stress or for reasons related to our past, we have distorted thoughts about our surroundings or ourselves. Some of these thoughts or beliefs can be very distressful and affect our daily living.

Try to think of a belief or thought you have that might cause you stress or worry.

1. A thought or belief I hold that causes some stress and that often bothers me is:

_____

_____

_____

2a Because of this thought or belief, I often feel

_____

_____

_____

2b Because of this thought or belief, I will

_____

_____

_____

3a What are the facts that support my thought or belief? *(Name at least three)*

_____

_____

_____

3b Have all these facts been checked?

_____

_____

_____

4. Try finding at least one alternative explanation for each fact.

_____

_____

_____

Together, we will look at our thoughts and beliefs and try to offer each other alternative explanations and suggestions for investigating facts.

What I wish to remember:

_____

_____

_____

_____

T-6: Looking at things from a positive perspective

Whether we attribute our success to talent or to luck, and see our mistakes as traits or isolated events makes all the difference. Our attributions will determine how we go through life: with optimism or pessimism. Today, we will look at how to have a positive outlook by changing attributions.

Lisa got an "A" on an exam...

A) *If her reaction was: "I got lucky" or "The teacher was probably feeling lenient" it would mean that Lisa experiences*

positive things = outside attributions

B) *If her reaction was: "I did great!" or "I studied well and it paid off" it would mean that Lisa experiences*

positive things = self attributions

John was driving his car in the rain and had an accident.

C) *If his reaction was: "I'm such a lousy driver!" or "I'm too absent-minded to drive in the rain" it would mean that John experiences*

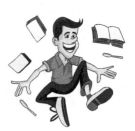

negative things = self attributions

D) *If his reaction was: "It's dangerous to drive in the rain" or "It was an accident, it can happen to anyone" it would mean that John experiences*

negative things = outside attributions

1. Which two reactions (A-B-C-D) do you think can make someone feel depressed or have a low self-esteem in the long run?

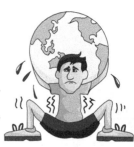

_____

_____

2. Which two reactions (A-B-C-D) do you think can make someone feel positive or have a higher self-esteem in the long run?

_____

_____

3. a) Think of a positive thing you experienced and write a statement that would be considered a *positive self attribution*.

_____

_____

   b) Think of a negative thing you experienced and write a statement that would be considered a *negative outside attribution*.

_____

_____

Situation (a)	Positive self attribution

Situation (b)	Negative outside attribution

What I wish to remember:

_____

_____

_____

_____

Homework: Fill out the "Positive Thinking" sheet in the Annex with other examples from your week.

What we learned and remember about Testing hypotheses and looking for alternatives:

1. _____

_____

_____

2. _____

_____

_____

3. _____

_____

_____

4. _____

_____

_____

5. _____

_____

_____

DRUGS, ALCOHOL AND HOW I FEEL

Learning objectives:

After having completed the activities in this section, each participant should be able to achieve or complete the following objectives:

1. The participant is able to identify him/herself in positive terms and name as least two values he/she shares with others in the group.
2. The participant is able to identify how drugs and alcohol can affect someone's reasoning, feelings and identity.
3. The participant is able to name at least two positive and effective ways to cope with feelings of depression or anxiety.

Activities:

D-1:	Words that describe me
D-2:	What I value
D-3:	Drugs and alcohol: when, where and with whom
D-4:	Their effect on my life
D-5:	Feeling down or hopeless
D-6:	Changing my mood

D-1: Words that describe me

It is often easier to recall our faults or negative qualities than our positive qualities. Today we will focus on the latter and discuss the importance of recognizing our positive qualities.

Circle the words that best describe you and write them on the poster-sheet with your name, on the wall.

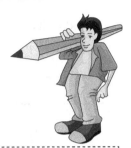

Sensitive	Confident	Sensible
Cool	Artistic	Nice to others
Helpful	Responsible	Healthy
Expressive	Independent	Energetic
Creative	Enthusiastic	Curious
Brave	Organised	Happy
Honest	Hardworking	Athletic
Leader	Kind	Resourceful
Good listener	Good team spirit	Good friend

Once you have finished copying your answers onto your poster sheet, look at the other participants' poster sheets, and add one or two positive qualities that you know about them but that they did not write down. You can write qualities that were not on the list.

Take a moment to look at the qualities on your poster sheet.

1. How does it feel to see words on your poster sheet, all describing something about you?

   _____

   _____

   _____

2. Which qualities written by others surprise you?

   _____

   _____

   _____

3. Which qualities make you really happy to see written?

   _____

   _____

   _____

4. Why is it important to remember these positive qualities about yourself?

   _____

   _____

   _____

Together, we will recall how it feels to have positive qualities that are appreciated by others and why it's important to remember these qualities to maintain a healthy self-esteem.

What I wish to remember:

_____

_____

_____

_____

D-2: What I value

Our values often determine our behavior ... we often refuse to do something that goes against them. Today, we are going to discuss our values, and see how they are similar or different. We will then review what was said, what we want to remember and what values we share.

Put a check to indicate how important each statement is for you. Compare your answers with the person on your right. We will then ask who marked "very important" or "important" beside each statement so we can see how many of us share similar values.

	Very important	Important	Not important
Being appreciated by others	_____	_____	_____
Being a good worker or student	_____	_____	_____
Spending time with family	_____	_____	_____
Expressing myself artistically	_____	_____	_____
Feeling good about myself	_____	_____	_____
Having a best friend	_____	_____	_____
Being respected by others	_____	_____	_____
Having fun	_____	_____	_____
Having money	_____	_____	_____
Being liked by teacher or boss	_____	_____	_____
Being proud of myself	_____	_____	_____
Being alone	_____	_____	_____
Looking good	_____	_____	_____
Spending time in nature	_____	_____	_____
Being popular	_____	_____	_____
Having time to do what I like	_____	_____	_____
Working out (exercising)	_____	_____	_____
Helping others if I can	_____	_____	_____
Being part of a group	_____	_____	_____
Other: _____	_____	_____	_____
_____	_____	_____	_____
_____	_____	_____	_____

Try to note who in the group, and how many people in the group, share the same values and interests as you.

What I wish to remember:

_____

_____

_____

_____

Homework of the week: Fill out another Goal sheet in the Annex, thinking of interests to develop, qualities to use or positive thinking skills.

D-3: Drugs and alcohol: when, where and with whom

Most of us have a drink or some type of drug from time to time, either in a social context or when trying to deal with negative emotions. Today, we are going to try to pinpoint those moments to help us better know ourselves.

Think back at the last 3 months and answer the following questions.

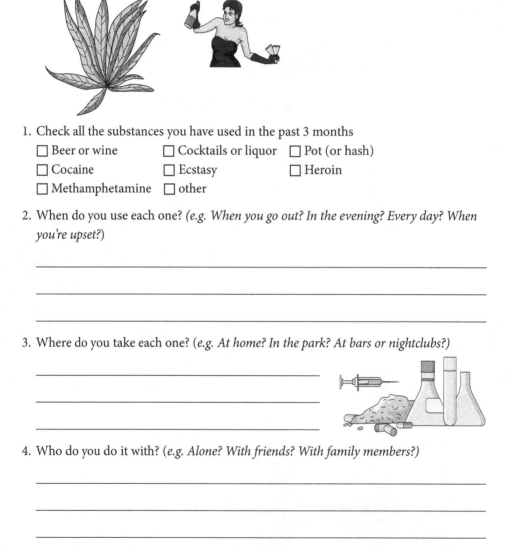

1. Check all the substances you have used in the past 3 months
   - ☐ Beer or wine
   - ☐ Cocktails or liquor
   - ☐ Pot (or hash)
   - ☐ Cocaine
   - ☐ Ecstasy
   - ☐ Heroin
   - ☐ Methamphetamine
   - ☐ other

2. When do you use each one? *(e.g. When you go out? In the evening? Every day? When you're upset?)*

   _____

   _____

   _____

3. Where do you take each one? *(e.g. At home? In the park? At bars or nightclubs?)*

   _____

   _____

   _____

4. Who do you do it with? *(e.g. Alone? With friends? With family members?)*

   _____

   _____

   _____

5. Are you worried about your use of one or more of the substances mentioned? If yes, what's worrying you?

_____

_____

_____

What I wish to remember:

_____

_____

_____

_____

> *Together, we will review the specific situations that might bring each of us to use drugs and alcohol in order to better understand our behavior, and modify it if needed.*

D-4: Their effect on my life

Drugs and alcohol used frequently or in excess can greatly impact most aspects of our lives. Today, we will look at how drugs and alcohol affect us and what we can do about it.

Check all the answers that apply to you

1. When I drink a lot, smoke pot or take some other drug,
   - ☐ a) immediately in a great mood but it doesn't last
   - ☐ b) very relaxed
   - ☐ c) a bit paranoid or aggressive
   - ☐ d) sad or depressed
   - ☐ e) cool, like I fit in with others
   - ☐ f) don't know, it's never happened to me
   - ☐ g) other:_____

2. The morning after I drank a lot or used drugs, I usually feel...
   - ☐ a) horrible... hungover (headache, a bit sick)
   - ☐ b) down, depressed, not wanting to get out of bed
   - ☐ c) slow, a bit confused
   - ☐ d) great, no problem, like a million bucks!
   - ☐ e) don't know, it's never happened to me
   - ☐ f) other:_____

3. In the long run, if I continue using alcohol or drugs frequently, I might...
   - ☐ a) have trouble in school or in keeping a job
   - ☐ b) develop health problems related to my drinking or drug habit
   - ☐ c) become poor from trying to support the habit
   - ☐ d) develop memory deficits and trouble concentrating
   - ☐ e) increase my stress level and have a psychotic relapse
   - ☐ f) alienate people around me
   - ☐ g) no problem, I don't drink or take drugs
   - ☐ h) other_____

4. If I wanted to diminish or stop my alcohol or drug consumption, I could...

☐ a) change friends, if they were my drinking or drug buddies

☐ b) avoid hanging out at places where I would usually consume

☐ c) try other ways to make myself feel better (e.g. exercise, arts, movies, relaxation)

☐ d) learn to say NO and be assertive about what I want in life

☐ e) join a support group (live or internet) to help me quit

☐ f) find someone to talk to when I feel tempted or down

☐ g) do nothing, I don't drink or take drugs

☐ h) other_____

DANGER
KEEP OUT

What I wish to remember:

_____

_____

_____

_____

Homework: Fill out a new Goal of the week sheet in the Annex, thinking of drugs or alcohol if it applies, using the "Drugs and Alcohol" sheet of the Annex to help.

D-5: Feeling down or hopeless

Most of us feel overwhelmed or depressed at one time or another in our lives. For some, thoughts of "ending it" might be considered. This activity aims at finding hope in the future and reasons not to act upon these thoughts.

Role play- done by one of the group leaders

"I'm really depressed... I think I want kill myself . . . There's no reason for me to go on... My family probably thinks I'm a burden . . . I have been diagnosed with schizophrenia and the drugs they're giving me are making me gain weight . . . All this has made me miss classes and now I'm having trouble finishing the year . . . There's nothing to look forward to, I should die . . ."

1. What questions might you ask that can make the person doubt that dying is the best choice? Go ahead, ask!

   _____

   _____

   _____

   _____

2. What might you say to convince that person that suicide is not the solution? Try it!

   _____

   _____

   _____

   _____

3. What can someone do to get out of that feeling of hopelessness?

   _____

   _____

   _____

   _____

4. Have you ever had suicidal ideas? If yes, what did you do to feel better?

   _____

   _____

   _____

   _____

What I wish to remember:

_____

_____

_____

_____

D-6: Changing my mood

Being able to find ways to feel better when we are feeling down or angry can at times be very difficult. Today we are going to try to find as many positive ways as possible to cope with such emotions. Take a few minutes to think about it, and we'll share our answers with the group.

1. a) When I'm feeling sad, down or depressed, what helps me is:

    _____

    _____

    _____

    _____

   b) One strategy (or more) that someone mentioned that could work for me is:

    _____

    _____

    _____

    _____

2. a) When I'm feeling angry, frustrated or aggressive, what helps me is:

    _____

    _____

    _____

    _____

   b) One strategy (or more) that someone mentioned that could work for me is:

    _____

    _____

    _____

    _____

What I wish to remember:

_____

_____

_____

_____

Homework: Try at least one of the suggestions made by another group member this week and check if it worked for you or not.

What we learned and remember about Drugs, alcohol and how I feel:

1. _____

_____

_____

2. _____

_____

_____

3. _____

_____

_____

4. _____

_____

_____

5. _____

_____

_____

COPING AND COMPETENCE

Learning objectives:

After having completed the activities in this section, each participant should be able to attain or complete the following objectives:

1. The participant is able to describe at least two techniques that help him/her relax or diminish symptoms.
2. The participant is able to identify which coping strategy works best for him/her in specific situations.
3. The participant can describe what he/she learned, achieved and improved since the beginning of the groups.

Activities:

C-1:   Relief from stress

C-2:   Dealing with symptoms

C-3:   Available resources

C-4:   My strengths, protective factors and challenges

C-5:   Coping my own way

C-6:   Review of the module

C-1: Relief from stress

Being able to find ways to calm down when we are stressed or preventing stress from over-coming us isn't always easy. Let's name and practice ways to deal with stress so we feel more in control with our lives.

Sometimes, we feel stressed out, agitated and it is diffi-cult to find a way to solve our problems. Is there a solu-tion to what is happening? When my body, my mind and my emotions are agitated by stress, my productivity or activity levels crash, which is why it is important to find a way to calm down.

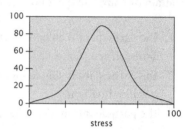

Yet, a certain amount of stress is important to stay active and productive. We want to learn to cope with enough stress to be active without increasing our symptoms.

We will try a relaxation exercise to calm down. This exercise won't solve your problems, but could help you to look at problems in a more peaceful state of mind. Let's try "Shavasan" a breathing exercise helpful to get rid of the tension associated with stress.

SHAVASAN

If done every day, this exercise is very efficient in relieving tension associated with stress. Done in a quiet environment—when you feel like you need it—it can help to take a break from what is worrying you.

1. *Lie with your back on the mattress, your arms outstretched, and legs wide apart, breathe out all the air from your lungs a few times.*

2. *Breathe air very slowly, filling your lungs from the bottom to the top. It is not a usual way to breathe, so keep concentrated on this specific way of breathing. Raise your stomach a little, but not as much as a balloon.*

3. *Breathe out, emptying your lungs from the top to the bottom. While the air comes out of your mouth, feel your body becoming heavier. Realize that with the air coming out, stress is following, going out of your whole body. If you feel a higher tension in a part of your body, let this tension go out with each exhale.*

4. *When your breathing becomes slow, calm and regular, make a little pause when all the air is exhaled from your lungs before inhaling, and breathe slowly after the pause, filling your lungs from the bottom to the top. When your lungs are filled with air, take another pause before breathing out.*

5. *Now, each time your lungs are emptied, say in your mind "RELAX," and breathe slowly. Do it a few times, until you feel very comfortable. You can also say "Shavasan" instead of "Relax," if you prefer.*

6. *If some thoughts are in your mind or are bothering you, identify these thoughts and let them go, concentrating on the way you breathe, slowly, regularly, saying "Relax" in your mind when your lungs are emptied.*

7. *When you feel the relief from tension, open your eyes and stand up slowly, experiencing the calm in your body, your mind and emotions.*

As a group, we will discuss the effects of Shavasan on the body, on the mind and on emotions.

What I wish to remember:

_____

_____

_____

_____

C-2: Dealing with symptoms

At times, symptoms can bother us more and we need to find ways to deal with them and stay well. Today, we will look at ways of dealing with distressing or annoying symptoms in order to feel better.

Different strategies can be used to deal with different symptoms. Sometimes, a strategy doesn't work and we need to try another until we are relieved from our symptom or we feel better and in control.

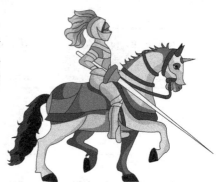

1. When I experience the symptom _____

   what usually helps me is _____

   if that doesn't work, I try _____

   if things seem to be getting worse I will _____

   _____

   One thing that doesn't help me is _____

   _____

2. When I start having the disturbing thought of _____

   _____

   what usually helps me is _____

   if that doesn't work, I try _____

   if really things seem to be getting worse I will _____

   _____

   One thing that doesn't help me is _____

   _____

3. Of the following list of possible coping strategies, circle all those you have tried before to deal with your symptoms or thoughts and made you feel better, check (✓) those you would want to try in the next two weeks and cross out those that you are sure would not help you.

Thoughts	Behaviors
☐ concentrate on the type of voice, tone, male or female, etc.	☐ take a hot bath or shower
☐ think of something positive or nice about myself	☐ have a massage
	☐ try relaxing techniques
☐ try to think of why I'm thinking this, what are the antecedents, what's the situation and what are the consequences of my thoughts on how I feel and behave	☐ listen to music
	☐ watch television
	☐ take a walk
	☐ exercise (sport)
	☐ humming or singing
	☐ speak to myself
☐ try to assess if I'm perceiving things right by checking for evidence	☐ call a friend to talk
	☐ go see a movie
☐ remind myself that even if my thoughts are scary, the situation is not really that bad or dangerous	☐ read a book or magazine
	☐ play a game
	☐ go on the internet
☐ Try to see things from a positive perspective by changing the attributions I make	☐ clean my room
	☐ go check for evidence for my beliefs
	☐ ask people I trust if my beliefs make sense and if they can hear the same voices
☐ forgive myself for wrongdoing	
☐ give myself pats on the back to encourage myself	☐ write diary of my emotions and daily thoughts
☐ tell myself that I have resources I can use to overcome my symptoms	☐ call my physician, case-manager or nurse to make an appointment
	☐ take my meds regularly
☐ accept myself with strengths and challenges	☐ participate in group meetings or activities
	☐ do something with my hands (crafts, drawings,...)
☐ try thinking and considering every possible alternative for my belief	
☐ try thinking of something else	

What I wish to remember:

_____

_____

_____

_____

Homework: Try one or more of the coping strategies listed in the Annex under "Coping strategies" and note which ones worked for you.

C-3: Available resources

It is important to know who you can count on and where you can get help when needed. Some people can give you information, some can give you emotional support or others can offer material support.

Information is an important type of support. It helps identify the "5 W's":

Who, what, where, when and why.

1. Think of who, in each of these categories, can provide informational support to you regarding your symptoms and overall well-being. Write each person's name down.

   In my family: _____

   My friend(s) _____

   Acquaintances _____

   Health professionals _____

   Community support groups _____

   Others _____

Emotional support is often needed in times of distress. It is found in people who listen to you, give you comfort, understanding and guidance.

2. Think of who, in each of these categories, can provide emotional support to you when you are not feeling well. Write each person's name down.

   In my family: _____

   My friend(s) _____

   Acquaintances _____

   Health professionals _____

   Community support groups _____

   Others _____

Material support is the type of support found when a person concretely helps you doing something you can't do by yourself. For example, someone giving you money, showing you how to do something or accompanying you in doing it.

3. Think of who, in each of these categories, can provide material support when you need it. Write each person's name down.

In my family: _____

My friend(s) _____

Acquaintances _____

Health professionals_____

Community support groups _____

Others _____

4. Who, among the people you listed, is someone that you trust enough to talk about your symptoms to and who could help you deal with stress or remind you of coping strategies when needed?

_____

_____

At the end of the group, you will receive a list of community support programs and other community resources that can be useful to you.

What I wish to remember:

_____

_____

_____

_____

Homework: Fill-out the "telephone resource list" provided to you in the Annex section so you will have the numbers handy.

C-4: My strengths, protective factors, and challenges

Think of your strengths, protective factors, and challenges and how they have changed. Answer the following questions. As a group, together we will observe if we have become more competent individuals.

1. What do you consider your strengths to be?

_____

_____

_____

2. What are your protective factors?

_____

_____

_____

3. What are your problems or difficulties?

_____

_____

_____

4. How will you go about overcoming these problems?

_____

_____

_____

5. In what do you consider having improved yourself?

_____

_____

_____

> *At the end, we will review the vulnerability-stress-competence model and see how our strengths and protective factors can help us deal with our symptoms and challenges in order to become more competent individuals.*

Review:

VULNERABILITY STRESS COMPETENCE MODEL

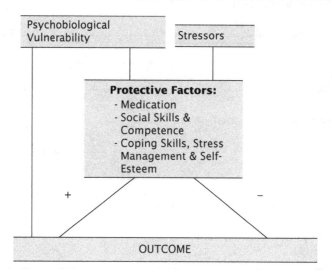

What I wish to remember:

_____

_____

_____

_____

Homework: Go back to the " Effectsof Stress" sheet in the Annex and check all the effects you experienced BEFORE you first started having symptoms or strange thoughts.

C-5: Coping my own way

Now that you have tried different coping strategies for controlling your symptoms and diminishing stress, we will look at what works better for you. We will make a staying well plan so you can continue being in control of your life.

1. On a daily basis, in order to stay well I will tell myself

_____

_____

_____

2. On a daily basis, in order to stay well I will

_____

_____

_____

3. In order to meet my long-term goals while staying well I must tell myself

_____

_____

_____

4. In order to meet my long-term goals while staying well I must

_____

_____

_____

5. I know things start going wrong before my symptoms get worse when I am experiencing the following (*refer to pages 10 to 13*):

_____

_____

_____

6. When things aren't going so well, either because I'm experiencing high levels of stress, my symptoms are getting worse or I'm very depressed, I should tell myself

_____

_____

_____

7. When things aren't going so well, either because I'm experiencing high levels of stress, my symptoms are getting worse or I'm very depressed, I should

_____

_____

_____

Together, we will discuss what helps us daily and in the long run. We will also see why a healthy self-esteem and a positive outlook are important ingredients in staying well.

What I wish to remember:

_____

_____

_____

_____

Homework: Share this Staying Well Plan with someone you trust from your support network and ask that person to make a copy of it to help you in the future, if needed.

C-6: Review of the module

We did it!!! We have covered the entire CBT module!!! As a group, together we will look at what we just experienced, what we learned, what we liked and what we didn't like as much. We will also look back at what we most want to remember about our group meetings.

1. What went particularly well for you during the meetings?

_____

_____

_____

2. What did you specifically like about the group meetings?

_____

_____

_____

3. What didn't you like?

_____

_____

_____

4. Who did you get to know better during the meetings?

_____

_____

_____

5. What have you tried to accomplish that you hadn't tried before the group?

_____

_____

_____

6. What did you learn about yourself during the meetings?

_____

_____

_____

7. What do you wish to remember about this whole experience?

_____

_____

_____

8. What are you going to continue working on in the near future?

_____

_____

_____

CONGRATULATIONS!

You have completed the module!!

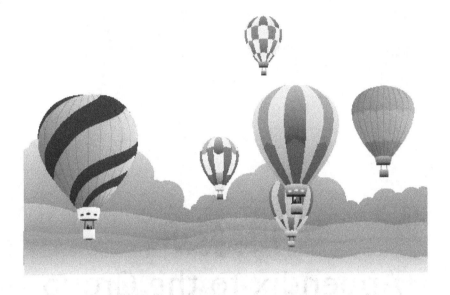

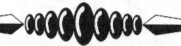

Appendix to the Group CBT for Psychosis Workbook

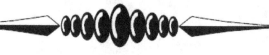

Effects of stress

Use this checklist to assess yourself regularly and verify the effects of stress on your body, mind and emotions.

The physical effects of stress (check all that apply to you now)

☐ My heartbeat is faster
☐ I can't fall asleep
☐ I wake up often during the night
☐ I sleep too much, more than usual
☐ I feel tired
☐ I feel weak
☐ I sweat more than usual
☐ My voice trembles
☐ I feel sick (nausea) or I throw up
☐ I am not hungry
☐ I can't stop eating
☐ Other: (describe)_____

☐ My cheeks turn red (blush)
☐ I turn pale
☐ My mouth is dry
☐ I feel aches all over my body
☐ My muscles become tense
☐ I constantly have to go to the bathroom
☐ I can't stop moving
☐ I can't stop doing the same thing over and over again
☐ I need to walk all the time
☐ I feel numb

The psychological effects of stress (check all that apply to you now)

☐ My ideas are speeding up
☐ The same thought keeps coming back
☐ I feel like I am trapped
☐ I don't know what to think
☐ I have doubts about everything
☐ I can't remember anything
☐ I can't get rid of a thought
☐ My ideas are not clear
☐ I want to forget everything
☐ Other: (describe)_____

☐ I am too excited and I can't clear up my mind
☐ I am thinking about bad things
☐ I can't understand what is going on
☐ I can't get over a detail about the event and I am losing track of "the big picture"
☐ I can't concentrate
☐ I can't organize my thoughts

The emotional effects of stress (check all that apply to you now)

- ☐ I feel afraid
- ☐ I feel like hiding away, isolating myself from everyone
- ☐ I feel responsible for a situation I didn't cause
- ☐ I feel discouraged
- ☐ I don't want to do anything
- ☐ I can't calm down
- ☐ I don't care about my physical appearance or hygiene
- ☐ I want everything to stop
- ☐ I want to do something crazy
- ☐ I am angry
- ☐ Other: (describe)_____

- ☐ I want to hurt someone
- ☐ I want to disappear
- ☐ I don't want to talk to anyone
- ☐ I don't recognize myself
- ☐ I feel like dirt
- ☐ I can't trust my best friends
- ☐ I feel guilty
- ☐ I don't trust myself
- ☐ I want to solve a problem by acting aggressively against someone or something
- ☐ I feel I am losing control of myself

Effects of stress

Use this checklist to assess yourself regularly and verify the effects of stress on your body, mind and emotions.

The physical effects of stress (check all that apply to you now)

☐ My heartbeat is faster

☐ I can't fall asleep

☐ I wake up often during the night

☐ I sleep too much, more than usual

☐ I feel tired

☐ I feel weak

☐ I sweat more than usual

☐ My voice trembles

☐ I feel sick (nausea) or I throw up

☐ I am not hungry

☐ I can't stop eating

☐ Other: (describe) _____

☐ My cheeks turn red (blush)

☐ I turn pale

☐ My mouth is dry

☐ I feel aches all over my body

☐ My muscles become tense

☐ I constantly have to go to the bathroom

☐ I can't stop moving

☐ I can't stop doing the same thing over and over again

☐ I need to walk all the time

☐ I feel numb

The psychological effects of stress (check all that apply to you now)

☐ My ideas are speeding up

☐ The same thought keeps coming back

☐ I feel like I am trapped

☐ I don't know what to think

☐ I have doubts about everything

☐ I can't remember anything

☐ I can't get rid of a thought

☐ My ideas are not clear

☐ I want to forget everything

☐ Other: (describe) _____

☐ I am too excited and I can't clear up my mind

☐ I am thinking about bad things

☐ I can't understand what is going on

☐ I can't get over a detail about the event and I am losing track of "the big picture"

☐ I can't concentrate

☐ I can't organize my thoughts

The emotional effects of stress (check all that apply to you now)

- ☐ I feel afraid
- ☐ I feel like hiding away, isolating myself from everyone
- ☐ I feel responsible for a situation I didn't cause
- ☐ I feel discouraged
- ☐ I don't want to do anything
- ☐ I can't calm down
- ☐ I don't care about my physical appearance or hygiene
- ☐ I want everything to stop
- ☐ I want to do something crazy
- ☐ I am angry
- ☐ Other: (describe)_____

- ☐ I want to hurt someone
- ☐ I want to disappear
- ☐ I don't want to talk to anyone
- ☐ I don't recognize myself
- ☐ I feel like dirt
- ☐ I can't trust my best friends
- ☐ I feel guilty
- ☐ I don't trust myself
- ☐ I want to solve a problem by acting aggressively against someone or something
- ☐ I feel I am losing control of myself

_____

Effects of stress

Use this checklist to assess yourself regularly and verify the effects of stress on your body, mind and emotions.

The physical effects of stress (check all that apply to you now)

☐ My heartbeat is faster
☐ I can't fall asleep
☐ I wake up often during the night
☐ I sleep too much, more than usual
☐ I feel tired
☐ I feel weak
☐ I sweat more than usual
☐ My voice trembles
☐ I feel sick (nausea) or throw up
☐ I am not hungry
☐ I can't stop eating

☐ My cheeks turn red (blush)
☐ I turn pale
☐ My mouth is dry
☐ I feel aches all over my body
☐ My muscles become tense
☐ I constantly have to go to the bathroom
☐ I can't stop moving
☐ I can't stop doing the same thing over and over again
☐ I need to walk all the time
☐ I feel numb

☐ Other: (describe)_____

_____

The psychological effects of stress (check all that apply to you now)

☐ My ideas are speeding up
☐ The same thought keeps coming back
☐ I think I am trapped
☐ I don't know what to think
☐ I have doubts about everything
☐ I can't remember anything
☐ I can't get rid of a thought
☐ My ideas are not clear
☐ I want to forget everything

☐ I am too excited and I can't clear up my mind
☐ I am thinking only about bad things
☐ I can't understand what is going on
☐ I can't get over a detail about the event and I am losing track of "the big picture"
☐ I can't concentrate
☐ I can't organize my thoughts

☐ Other: (describe)_____

_____

The emotional effects of stress (check all that apply to you now)

- ☐ I am afraid
- ☐ I feel like hiding away, isolating myself from everyone
- ☐ I am feeling responsible for a situation I didn't cause
- ☐ I am feeling discouraged
- ☐ I don't want to do anything
- ☐ I can't calm down
- ☐ I don't care about my physical appearance or hygiene
- ☐ I want it to stop right now
- ☐ I want to do something crazy
- ☐ I am angry
- ☐ Other: (describe)_____

- ☐ I want to hurt someone
- ☐ I want to disappear
- ☐ I don't want to talk to anyone
- ☐ I can't recognize myself
- ☐ I am feeling like dirt
- ☐ I can't trust my best friends
- ☐ I am feeling guilty
- ☐ I can't trust myself
- ☐ I am making plans to solve a problem by acting aggressively against someone or something
- ☐ I am losing control of myself

_____

Effects of stress

Use this checklist to assess yourself regularly and verify the effects of stress on your body, mind and emotions.

The physical effects of stress (check all that apply to you now)

☐ My heartbeat is faster
☐ I can't fall asleep
☐ I wake up often during the night
☐ I sleep too much, more than usual
☐ I feel tired
☐ I feel weak
☐ I sweat more than usual
☐ My voice trembles
☐ I feel sick (nausea) or I throw up
☐ I am not hungry
☐ I can't stop eating
☐ Other: (describe)_____

☐ My cheeks turn red (blush)
☐ I turn pale
☐ My mouth is dry
☐ I feel aches all over my body
☐ My muscles become tense
☐ I constantly have to go to the bathroom
☐ I can't stop moving
☐ I can't stop doing the same thing over and over again
☐ I need to walk all the time
☐ I feel numb

_____

The psychological effects of stress (check all that apply to you now)

☐ My ideas are speeding up
☐ The same thought keeps coming back
☐ I feel like I am trapped
☐ I don't know what to think
☐ I have doubts about everything
☐ I can't remember anything
☐ I can't get rid of a thought
☐ My ideas are not clear
☐ I want to forget everything
☐ Other: (describe)_____

☐ I am too excited and I can't clear up my mind
☐ I am thinking about bad things
☐ I can't understand what is going on
☐ I can't get over a detail about the event and I am losing track of "the big picture"
☐ I can't concentrate
☐ I can't organize my thoughts

_____

The emotional effects of stress (check all that apply to you now)

- ☐ I feel afraid
- ☐ I feel like hiding away, isolating myself from everyone
- ☐ I feel responsible for a situation I didn't cause
- ☐ I feel discouraged
- ☐ I don't want to do anything
- ☐ I can't calm down
- ☐ I don't care about my physical appearance or hygiene
- ☐ I want everything to stop
- ☐ I want to do something crazy
- ☐ I am angry
- ☐ Other: (describe)_____

- ☐ I want to hurt someone
- ☐ I want to disappear
- ☐ I don't want to talk to anyone
- ☐ I don't recognize myself
- ☐ I feel like dirt
- ☐ I can't trust my best friends
- ☐ I feel guilty
- ☐ I don't trust myself
- ☐ I want to solve a problem by acting aggressively against someone or something
- ☐ I feel I am losing control of myself

MY STRESS LEVEL

Take the time to rate your stress level in order to evaluate if you need to use coping or protective factors.

Level 0	**Feeling good** I am calm, at peace with myself.
Level 1	**Minimal stress** I feel a little nervous, or agitated. It is temporary and I don't mind.
Level 2	**Light stress** I feel a little discomfort and I am trying to understand what is going on.
Level 3	**Moderate stress** Effects on my body, mind and emotions, but I am still in control. I can go on.
Level 4	**Important stress** I feel strange, uncomfortable. My heart is pounding and my muscles are tense. I am trying to find out how to stay in control.
Level 5	**Anxiety** I don't breathe easily, I'm feeling strange, or dizzy. I am afraid I am going to lose control. I want to run away.
Level 6	**Moderate anxiety** My heart is pounding, I feel disoriented, like if it was not real. I can't breathe normally. I can't control myself any longer.
Level 7	**Panic** It is physically painful. I am afraid, I think I'm going to lose my mind. I am afraid of dying, I want to run away and escape right now.

MY STRESS LEVEL

Take the time to rate your stress level in order to evaluate if you need to use coping or protective factors.

Level 0	**Feeling good** I am calm, at peace with myself.
Level 1	**Minimal stress** I feel a little nervous, or agitated. It is temporary and I don't mind.
Level 2	**Light stress** I feel a little discomfort and I am trying to understand what is going on.
Level 3	**Moderate stress** Effects on my body, mind and emotions, but I am still in control. I can go on.
Level 4	**Important stress** I feel strange, uncomfortable. My heart is pounding and my muscles are tense. I am trying to find out how to stay in control.
Level 5	**Anxiety** I don't breathe easily, I'm feeling strange, or dizzy. I am afraid I am going to lose control. I want to run away.
Level 6	**Moderate anxiety** My heart is pounding, I feel disoriented, like if it was not real. I can't breathe normally. I can't control myself any longer.
Level 7	**Panic** It is physically painful. I am afraid, I think I'm going to lose my mind. I am afraid of dying, I want to run away and escape right now.

MY STRESS LEVEL

Take the time to rate your stress level in order to evaluate if you need to use coping or protective factors.

Level 0	**Feeling good** I am calm, at peace with myself.
Level 1	**Minimal stress** I feel a little nervous, or agitated. It is temporary and I don't mind.
Level 2	**Light stress** I feel a little discomfort and I am trying to understand what is going on.
Level 3	**Moderate stress** Effects on my body, mind and emotions, but I am still in control. I can go on.
Level 4	**Important stress** I feel strange, uncomfortable. My heart is pounding and my muscles are tense. I am trying to find out how to stay in control.
Level 5	**Anxiety** I don't breathe easily, I'm feeling strange, or dizzy. I am afraid I am going to lose control. I want to run away.
Level 6	**Moderate anxiety** My heart is pounding, I feel disoriented, like if it was not real. I can't breathe normally. I can't control myself any longer.
Level 7	**Panic** It is physically painful. I am afraid, I think I'm going to lose my mind. I am afraid of dying, I want to run away and escape right now.

MY STRESS LEVEL

Take the time to rate your stress level in order to evaluate if you need to use coping or protective factors.

Level 0	**Feeling good**
	I am calm, at peace with myself.
Level 1	**Minimal stress**
	I feel a little nervous, or agitated. It is temporary and I don't mind.
Level 2	**Light stress**
	I feel a little discomfort and I am trying to understand what is going on.
Level 3	**Moderate stress**
	Effects on my body, mind and emotions, but I am still in control.
	I can go on.
Level 4	**Important stress**
	I feel strange, uncomfortable. My heart is pounding
	and my muscles are tense. I am trying to find out how to stay in control.
Level 5	**Anxiety**
	I don't breathe easily, I'm feeling strange, or dizzy. I am afraid
	I am going to lose control. I want to run away.
Level 6	**Moderate anxiety**
	My heart is pounding, I feel disoriented, like if it was
	not real. I can't breathe normally. I can't control myself any longer.
Level 7	**Panic**
	It is physically painful. I am afraid, I think I'm going to lose my mind.
	I am afraid of dying, I want to run away and escape right now.

These *"Goals of the Week"* sheets are for you, so you can continue to set and meet your goals each week even if the group meetings are over.

Goals of the Week

date: _____

Day	Goal	Not met	Partly met	Met
Monday				
Tuesday				
Wednesday				
Thursday				
Friday				
Saturday				
Sunday				

Goals of the Week

date: _____

Day	Goal	Not met	Partly met	Met
Monday				
Tuesday				
Wednesday				
Thursday				
Friday				
Saturday				
Sunday				

Goals of the Week

date:_____

Day	Goal	Not met	Partly met	Met
Monday				
Tuesday				
Wednesday				
Thursday				
Friday				
Saturday				
Sunday				

Goals of the Week

date:_____

Day	Goal	Not met	Partly met	Met
Monday				
Tuesday				
Wednesday				
Thursday				
Friday				
Saturday				
Sunday				

Goals of the Week

date: _____

Day	Goal	Not met	Partly met	Met
Monday				
Tuesday				
Wednesday				
Thursday				
Friday				
Saturday				
Sunday				

Goals of the Week

date: _____

Day	Goal	Not met	Partly met	Met
Monday				
Tuesday				
Wednesday				
Thursday				
Friday				
Saturday				
Sunday				

Goals of the Week

date:_____

Day	Goal	Not met	Partly met	Met
Monday				
Tuesday				
Wednesday				
Thursday				
Friday				
Saturday				
Sunday				

Goals of the Week

date: _____

Day	Goal	Not met	Partly met	Met
Monday				
Tuesday				
Wednesday				
Thursday				
Friday				
Saturday				
Sunday				

Goals of the Week

date: _____

Day	Goal	Not met	Partly met	Met
Monday				
Tuesday				
Wednesday				
Thursday				
Friday				
Saturday				
Sunday				

Goals of the Week

date:_____

Day	Goal	Not met	Partly met	Met
Monday				
Tuesday				
Wednesday				
Thursday				
Friday				
Saturday				
Sunday				

Goals of the Week

date: _____

Day	Goal	Not met	Partly met	Met
Monday				
Tuesday				
Wednesday				
Thursday				
Friday				
Saturday				
Sunday				

Goals of the Week

date: _____

Day	Goal	Not met	Partly met	Met
Monday				
Tuesday				
Wednesday				
Thursday				
Friday				
Saturday				
Sunday				

Goals of the Week

date: _____

Day	Goal	Not met	Partly met	Met
Monday				
Tuesday				
Wednesday				
Thursday				
Friday				
Saturday				
Sunday				

Goals of the Week

date: _____

Day	Goal	Not met	Partly met	Met
Monday				
Tuesday				
Wednesday				
Thursday				
Friday				
Saturday				
Sunday				

Goals of the Week

date:_____

Day	Goal	Not met	Partly met	Met
Monday				
Tuesday				
Wednesday				
Thursday				
Friday				
Saturday				
Sunday				

ABC's of CBT

You have seen, heard or thought that something is going on and you are about to act upon it, take a minute to do the ABC, starting by B - your belief, then think of why you are thinking that (A) and what you want to do and how you feel (C).

A for Antecedent What's the situation	B for Belief What do I think is going on?	C for consequence 1) How do I feel? 2) What do I want to do?
Alternative:		1) 2)

Next check the facts... here are some questions that can help you:

Who did it happen to?

Where did it happen?

Was anyone else involved?

Any witnesses? If yes, what did they see or hear?

Has any such thing ever happened before?

Why did it happen to that person (or to me)?

How can I be 100% sure of these facts?

Are there any other possible explanations for the event?

If yes, what?

Then, write the same A (situation) but try to think of a different B, an alternative hypothesis, and how you could feel and act differently (C)

A for Antecedent What's the situation	B for Belief What do I think is going on?	C for consequence 1) How do I feel? 2) What do I want to do?
Alternative:		1) 2)

ABC's of CBT

You have seen, heard or thought that something is going on and you are about to act upon it, take a minute to do the ABC, starting by B - your belief, then think of why you are thinking that (A) and what you want to do and how you feel (C).

A for Antecedent What's the situation	B for Belief What do I think is going on?	C for consequence 1) How do I feel? 2) What do I want to do?
Alternative:		1) 2)

Next check the facts... here are some questions that can help you:

Who did it happen to?

Where did it happen?

Was anyone else involved?

Any witnesses? If yes, what did they see or hear?

Has any such thing ever happened before?

Why did it happen to that person (or to me)?

How can I be 100% sure of these facts?

Are there any other possible explanations for the event?

If yes, what?

Then, write the same A (situation) but try to think of a different B, an alternative hypothesis, and how you could feel and act differently (C)

A for Antecedent What's the situation	B for Belief What do I think is going on?	C for consequence 1) How do I feel? 2) What do I want to do?
Alternative:		1) 2)

ABC's of CBT

You have seen, heard or thought that something is going on and you are about to act upon it, take a minute to do the ABC, starting by B - your belief, then think of why you are thinking that (A) and what you want to do and how you feel (C).

A for Antecedent What's the situation	B for Belief What do I think is going on?	C for consequence 1) How do I feel? 2) What do I want to do?
Alternative:		1) 2)

Next check the facts... here are some questions that can help you:

Who did it happen to?

Where did it happen?

Was anyone else involved?

Any witnesses? If yes, what did they see or hear?

Has any such thing ever happened before?

Why did it happen to that person (or to me)?

How can I be 100% sure of these facts?

Are there any other possible explanations for the event?

If yes, what?

Then, write the same A (situation) but try to think of a different B, an alternative hypothesis, and how you could feel and act differently (C)

A for Antecedent What's the situation	B for Belief What do I think is going on?	C for consequence 1) How do I feel? 2) What do I want to do?
Alternative:		1) 2)

ABC's of CBT

You have seen, heard or thought that something is going on and you are about to act upon it, take a minute to do the ABC, starting by B - your belief, then think of why you are thinking that (A) and what you want to do and how you feel (C).

A for Antecedent What's the situation	B for Belief What do I think is going on?	C for consequence 1) How do I feel? 2) What do I want to do?
Alternative:		1) 2)

Next check the facts... here are some questions that can help you:

Who did it happen to?

Where did it happen?

Was anyone else involved?

Any witnesses? If yes, what did they see or hear?

Has any such thing ever happened before?

Why did it happen to that person (or to me)?

How can I be 100% sure of these facts?

Are there any other possible explanations for the event?

If yes, what?

Then, write the same A (situation) but try to think of a different B, an alternative hypothesis, and how you could feel and act differently (C)

A for Antecedent What's the situation	B for Belief What do I think is going on?	C for consequence 1) How do I feel? 2) What do I want to do?
Alternative:		1) 2)

Positive thinking

The way we see ourselves and our actions can greatly influence how we feel about life (optimistic or pessimistic).

Remember that an optimistic person with a strong self-esteem will tend to explain:

negative things = outside attributions

positive things = self attributions

You should practice this too . . .

a) Think of a positive thing you experienced and fill in the table with a ***positive self attribution***.

Situation (a)	Positive self attribution

b) Think of a negative thing you experienced and fill in the table with a ***negative outside attribution***.

Situation (b)	Negative outside attribution

Positive thinking

The way we see ourselves and our actions can greatly influence how we feel about life (optimistic or pessimistic).

Remember that an optimistic person with a strong self-esteem will tend to explain:

negative things = outside attributions

positive things = self attributions

You should practice this too...

a) Think of a positive thing you experienced and fill in the table with *a positive self attribution*.

Situation (a)	Positive self attribution

b) Think of a negative thing you experienced and fill in the table with *a negative outside attribution*.

Situation (b)	Negative outside attribution

Drugs and alcohol

Here's a reminder of how drugs and alcohol can impact your life in the long run and suggestions about how to stop.

Answer these questions once in a while if you fear your consumption is becoming a problem.

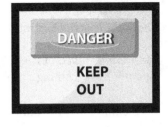

In the long run, if I continue using alcohol or drugs frequently, I might...

☐ a) have trouble in school or in keeping a job

☐ b) develop health problems related to my drinking or drug habit

☐ c) become poor from trying to support the habit

☐ d) develop memory deficits and trouble concentrating

☐ e) increase my stress level and have a psychotic relapse

☐ f) alienate people around me

☐ g) other_____

If I wanted to diminish or stop my alcohol or drug consumption, I could...

☐ a) change friends, if they're drinking or drug buddies

☐ b) avoid hanging out at places where I would usually consume

☐ c) try other ways to make myself feel better (e.g. exercise, arts, movies, relaxation)

☐ d) learn to say NO and be assertive about what I want in life

☐ e) join a support group (live or internet) to help me quit

☐ f) find someone to talk to when I feel tempted or down

☐ g) other _____

Drugs and alcohol

Here's a reminder of how drugs and alcohol can impact your life in the long run and suggestions about how to stop.

Answer these questions once in a while if you fear your consumption is becoming a problem.

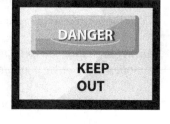

In the long run, if I continue using alcohol or drugs frequently, I might...

☐ a) have trouble in school or in keeping a job

☐ b) develop health problems related to my drinking or drug habit

☐ c) become poor from trying to support the habit

☐ d) develop memory deficits and trouble concentrating

☐ e) increase my stress level and have a psychotic relapse

☐ f) alienate people around me

☐ g) other_____

If I wanted to diminish or stop my alcohol or drug consumption, I could...

☐ a) change friends, if they're drinking or drug buddies

☐ b) avoid hanging out at places where I would usually consume

☐ c) try other ways to make myself feel better (e.g. exercise, arts, movies, relaxation)

☐ d) learn to say NO and be assertive about what I want in life

☐ e) join a support group (live or internet) to help me quit

☐ f) find someone to talk to when I feel tempted or down

☐ g) other_____

Coping strategies

Here's a list of coping strategies that are either related to your thoughts or to behaviors that can help you deal with symptoms. Take a look at it once in a while when you are looking for ways to feel better or to stay well.

Thoughts	Behaviors
☐ concentrate on the type of voice, tone, male or female, etc.	☐ take a hot bath or shower
☐ think of something positive or nice about myself	☐ have a massage
☐ try to think of why I'm thinking this, what are the antecedents, what's the situation and what are the consequences of my thoughts on how I feel and behave	☐ try relaxing techniques
	☐ listen to music
	☐ watch television
	☐ take a walk
	☐ exercise (sport)
	☐ humming or singing
	☐ speak to myself
☐ try to assess if I'm perceiving things right by checking for evidence	☐ call a friend to talk
☐ remind myself that even if my thoughts are scary, the situation is not really that bad or dangerous	☐ go see a movie
	☐ read a book or magazine
	☐ play a game
☐ Try to see things from a positive perspective by changing the attributions I make	☐ go on the internet
	☐ clean my room
	☐ go check for evidence for my beliefs
☐ forgive myself for wrongdoing	☐ ask people I trust if my beliefs make sense and if they can hear the same voices
☐ give myself pats on the back to encourage myself	
☐ tell myself that I have resources I can use to overcome my symptoms	☐ write diary of my emotions and daily thoughts
☐ accept myself with strengths and challenges	☐ call my physician, case-manager or nurse to make an appointment
	☐ take my meds regularly
☐ try thinking and considering every possible alternative for my belief	☐ participate in group meetings or activities
☐ try thinking of something else	☐ do something with my hands (crafts, drawings...)

Telephone resource list

Fill out the following:

People I can count on for **informational support**, people who can give me information that is helpful regarding my symptoms or my health (think of family, friends, acquaintances, health professionals, community groups, etc.):

Name_____ Phone number_____

Name_____ Phone number_____

Name_____ Phone number_____

Name_____ Phone number_____

Name_____ Phone number_____

People I can count on for **emotional support**, people who can listen to me or help me when I'm not feeling so well (think of family, friends, acquaintances, health professionals, community groups, etc.):

Name_____ Phone number_____

Name_____ Phone number_____

Name_____ Phone number_____

Name_____ Phone number_____

Name_____ Phone number_____

People I can count on for **material support**, people who can concretely give me tools when I need them (e.g. money, meds, show me how to do something) (think of family, friends, acquaintances, health professionals, community groups, etc.):

Name_____ Phone number_____

Name_____ Phone number_____

Name_____ Phone number_____

Name_____ Phone number_____

Name_____ Phone number_____

Community resources

Here is a list of resources available in your area. It is important that you know what is available if you wish to use any of these services. The group therapists will give you a list to insert here.

Example of a Diploma for the Graduation

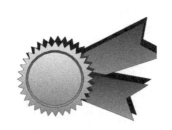

Date: _____

We hereby attest that _____ has successfully completed the training entitled: CBT.

Therapist name & signature

_____

Therapist name & signature

List of Sessions Used in Brief Inpatient Group CBT for Psychosis

Sessions Used for the Brief Inpatient 16-Session Format

S-1: Introducing ourselves
S-2: What is stress?
S-3: What do I consider stressful?
S-5: Vulnerability-stress-competence model

T-1: The ABC's of CBT
T-2: Common experiences
T-3: The traffic jam
T-4: How not-to-jump-to conclusions
T-5: Considering alternatives for my own beliefs

D-1: Words that describe me
D-6: Changing my mood

C-1: Relief from stress
C-2: Dealing with symptoms
C-3: Available resources
C-5: Coping my own way
C-6: Review of the module

Participation Scale

Participation Rating – CBT

Date : _____

Name of participant	Attention	Visual contact	Verbal participation	Questions	Help	Socialization	Disruptive behavior (-)	Confusion (-)	TOTAL
Total of group:									
Group average:									

Follow the scale legend for criteria

Signature of group therapists : _____ _____

Scale for the CBTp Participation Rating Scale (Leclerc, 1998)

For each item, use the following scores:

0   **means the absence of the behavior.**

1   **means a slight presence of the behavior**

2   **means the moderate presence of the behavior**

3   **means the strong presence of the behavior**

4   **means the exceptional presence of the behavior**

ATTENTION

For ATTENTION, 0 means the person was not paying attention at all during the session, 1 means low attention, 2 means moderate (half the time seemed present), 3 means fairly good attention (only missing short parts of the session or talks), and 4 means person stayed attentive throughout the session.

VISUAL CONTACT

For VISUAL CONTACT, 0 means the person wasn't making eye contact with anyone during the session, 1 means a few short looks, 2 means would look at people half the time (otherwise stare at book or elsewhere), 3 means a good visual contact (looking at people while speaking and only rarely looking elsewhere when others were talking), and 4 means kept eye contact throughout the session.

VERBAL PARTICIPATION

For VERBAL PARTICIPATION, 0 means the person did not say a word during the session, 1 means the person spoke at least once even if prompted to, 2 means the person spoke a few times even if prompted to, 3 means the person spoke regularly though not always prompted, and 4 means the person was actively verbally engaged throughout the session.

QUESTIONS

For QUESTIONS, 0 means no questions were asked by the person during the session, 1 means at least one question was asked at one moment during the session, 2 means at least two questions were asked with or without prompting, 3 means regular questions were asked, and 4 means the person asked many relevant questions during the session.

HELP

For HELP, 0 means the person hasn't tried to help anyone during the session, 1 means at least one offer to help, 2 means a few helpful offers or behaviors during the session, 3 means the person offered help and was helpful few times during the session, and 4 means the person is definitely very helpful to others in the group.

SOCIALIZATION

For SOCIALIZATION, 0 means no attempts to socialize whatsoever during the social break (person might leave early, not talk, etc.), 1 means the person tried at least once to socialize even if prompted, 2 means the person socialized a bit even if prompted, 3 means the person was somewhat sociable, and 4 means the person was very sociable, asked questions and seemed interested in others.

DISRUPTIVE BEHAVIOR: (NEGATIVE SCORE)

Disruptive behaviors are all behaviors that disrupt the good functioning of the group such as aggressive, nonempathic, nonrespectful, or monopolizing the discussion. A 0 means a total absence disruptive behaviors, a 1 means a mild disruption caused by the person, a 2 means a few disruptive behaviors (irrelevant jokes, for instance), 3 means many or more important disruptive behaviors (person is intoxicated and is constantly fooling around), and 4 means important disruptive behaviors (insults, shouting, etc.) necessitating the removal of the person from the group.

CONFUSION: (NEGATIVE SCORE)

This score assesses incoherence, rambling incomprehensively, tangentially, etc. A 0 means the person is not confused at all, a 1 means the person said one thing or sentence that was confusing but could vaguely explain it, a 2 means the person said a few things that suggested confusion, a 3 means the person is quite confused and really hard to understand, and a 4 means the person couldn't make sense or speak coherently throughout the session.

TOTAL: Add all the lines up to socialization and subtract the disruptive behavior and confusion score for each person

Self-Esteem Rating Scale—Short Form

(Lecomte, Corbière, & Laisné, 2006)

Name_____   ID #_____

This questionnaire is designed to measure how you feel about yourself. It is not a test, so there are no right or wrong answers. Please answer each item carefully and as accurately as you can by using the following scale:

   1 = Never
   2 = Rarely
   3 = A little of the time
   4 = Some of the time
   5 = A good part of the time
   6 = Most of the time
   7 = Always

1. __* I feel that others do things much better than I do.
2. __ I feel confident in my ability to deal with people.
3. __* I feel that I am likely to fail at things I do.
4. __ I feel that people really like to talk with me.
5. __ I feel that I am a very competent person.
6. __ When I am with other people, I feel that they are glad I am with them.
7. __ I feel that I make a good impression on others.

8. __ I feel confident that I can begin new relationships if I want to.
9. __* I feel ashamed about myself.
10. __* I feel inferior to other people.
11. __ I feel that my friends find me interesting.
12. __ I feel that I have a good sense of humor.
13. __* I get angry at myself over the way I am.
14. __ My friends value me a lot.
15. __* I am afraid I will appear stupid to others.
16. __* I wish I could just disappear when I am around other people.
17. __* I feel that if I could be more like other people then I would feel better about myself.
18. __* I feel that I get pushed around more than others.
19. __ I feel that people have a good time when they are with me.
20. __* I wish that I were someone else.

First Episode Social Functioning Scale—Self-Report

(Lecomte, Corbière, Lehman, et al., 2013)

Please answer each question honestly, using the choices suggested.
If you answer Never, or if you find a question doesn't apply to you and answer N/A,
please explain why.

1. Living skills

1.1 Transportation

1.1.A I can get around town easily, either by taking the bus or by other means of transportation.

Totally Disagree   Disagree   Agree   Totally Agree

1.1.B In the past 3 months, I have used public transit or other means of transportation (car, bike etc.) to get around.

Never   Sometimes   Often   Always   N/A
(less than once a   (once a week)   (several x's/week)   (almost daily)
month)

If N/A or Never, please explain: (e.g., lack of resources, no need)

_____

_____

1.2 Communication

1.2.A I am comfortable using the phone, internet, or email to communicate.

Totally Disagree   Disagree   Agree   Totally Agree

1.2.B In the past 3 months, I have used the phone, internet, or email to communicate with people.

Never   Sometimes   Often   Always   N/A
(less than once a   (once a week)   (several x's/week)   (almost daily)
month)

If N/A or Never, please explain: (e.g., no need)

_____

_____

1.3 Basic hygiene

1.3.A I am good at taking care of my physical appearance and hygiene.

Totally Disagree   Disagree   Agree   Totally Agree

1.3.B In the past 3 months, I have been taking care of my appearance and hygiene.

Never   Sometimes   Often   Always   N/A
(shower once/week   (shower every 2–3   (shower   (always clean,
or less)   days, clothes can   almost daily)   shower daily)
be dirty)

If N/A or Never, please explain: (e.g., lack of energy, no motivation)

_____

_____

1.4 Getting food

1.4.A I have no problem getting enough food to eat (by cooking, family, fast food, etc.).

Totally Disagree   Disagree   Agree   Totally Agree

1.4.B In the past 3 months, I have been getting enough food to eat.

Never (always hungry)	Sometimes (skip meals, don't eat enough)	Often (usually well fed)	Always (eat 2–3 good meals per day)	N/A

If N/A or Never, please explain: (e.g., lack of resources, not hungry)

_____

_____

On a scale of 1 to 10, overall how important is it for you to be good in the areas of your daily living skills just mentioned (use of transportation, use of communication devices, basic hygiene, getting food)?

1 2 3 4 5 6 7 8 9 10
(not at all important)   (extremely important)

Comments: _____

_____

_____

2. Interacting with people

2.1 CLERKS, COFFEE SHOP. . .

2.1.A I find it easy to interact with waiters, cashiers, and salespeople (e.g., small talk, asking for information, making a purchase).

Totally Disagree	Disagree	Agree	Totally Agree

2.1.B In the past 3 months, I have been interacting with waiters, cashiers or salespeople.

Never (don't go near stores)	Sometimes (once or twice/month)	Often (more than once/ week)	Always (most days)	N/A

If N/A or Never, please explain: (e.g., not interested, no need)

_____

_____

2.2 Authority/ adults

2.2.A I find it easy to interact with authority figures (e.g. teacher, boss, doctor, others' parents . . .).

Totally Disagree   Disagree   Agree   Totally Agree

2.2.B In the past 3 months, I have been interacting with authority figures.

Never   Sometimes   Often   Always   N/A
(don't)   (less than once a week)   (most days)   (every day)

If N/A or Never, please explain: (e.g., no contact with authority figures)

_____

_____

2.3 Acquaintances

2.3.A I find it easy to talk with people my age I know just a little bit.

Totally Disagree   Disagree   Agree   Totally Agree

2.3.B In the past 3 months, I have been talking to people my age I know just a little bit.

Never   Sometimes   Often   Always   N/A
(don't)   (less than once a month)   (at least once a week)   (most days)

If N/A or Never, please explain: (e.g., no interest)

_____

_____

2.4 Assertiveness

2.4.A I know how to stand up for myself when needed.

Totally Disagree   Disagree   Agree   Totally Agree

2.4.B In the past 3 months, I have been able to stand up for myself.

Never   Sometimes   Often   Always   N/A
              (less than weekly) (most days)   (every day)

If N/A or Never, please explain: (e.g., no need to)

_____

_____

On a scale of 1 to 10, how important is it for you to be good in the areas of interacting with people just mentioned (interacting with waiters, authority figures, and acquaintances, and being assertive)?

              1   2   3   4   5   6   7   8   9   10
        (not at all important)   (extremely important)

Comments:_____

_____

_____

3. Friends and activities

3.1 SOLO ACTIVITIES

3.1.A I am really good in solo activities such as going to the gym, going to the movies, chatting on the net, taking lessons (music, painting, etc.). Please do not count watching TV, listening to music, or playing video games.

Totally Disagree   Disagree   Agree   Totally Agree

3.1.B In the past 3 months, I have been doing solo activities such as going to the gym, going to the movies, chatting on the net, taking lessons (music, painting, etc.).

Never   Sometimes   Often   Always   N/A
(don't)   (less than once a (several times a   (a few times/week)
             month)   month)

If N/A or Never, please explain: (e.g., too busy, no interest)

_____

_____

3.2 Meaningful activities

3.2.A I try to do things that are really important to me (specific hobbies, passions...).

Totally Disagree   Disagree   Agree   Totally Agree

3.2.B In the past 3 months, I have been doing things that are really important to me.

Never (don't)	Sometimes (less than once a month)	Often (several times a month)	Always (a few times/week)	N/A

If N/A or Never, please explain: (e.g., too busy, no hobbies)

_____

_____

3.3 Balancing time alone and with others

3.3.A I am able to balance the amount of time I spend with others and by myself.

Totally Disagree   Disagree   Agree   Totally Agree

3.3.B In the past 3 months, I have been spending most of my days alone.

Never	Sometimes (a few days a week)	Often (most days)	Always (every day)	N/A

If N/A or Never, please explain: (e.g., live with people, too busy)

_____

_____

3.4 Best friend

3.4.A I feel I have at least one best friend with whom I can share important things that happen to me.

Totally Disagree   Disagree   Agree   Totally Agree

3.4.B In the past 3 months, I have spent time with my best friend (live or by phone).

Never	Sometimes (spoke at least once)	Often (speak or see every 2–3 weeks)	Always (speak or see weekly)	N/A

If N/A or Never, please explain: (e.g., no best friend, too busy)

_____

_____

3.5 BUDDIES

3.5.A I have friends that I can hang out with, do stuff with (shopping, movies, go out . . .).

Totally Disagree   Disagree   Agree   Totally Agree

3.5.B In the past 3 months, I have spent time doing activities with my friends.

Never	Sometimes (at least once a month)	Often (several times a month)	Always (weekly)	N/A

If N/A or Never, please explain: (e.g., no money, too busy)

_____

_____

3.6 ABILITIES TO DEVELOP FRIENDSHIPS

3.6.A I am able to make new friends by suggesting getting together, making invitations, or phoning people up.

Totally Disagree   Disagree   Agree   Totally Agree

3.6.B In the past 3 months, I have tried to develop a potential friendship with someone.

Never	Sometimes (made an invitation or accepted one)	Often (invited, suggested activity, or did something with a new person more than once)	Always (very sociable, talk to new people, and open to meeting 3x's or more)	N/A

If N/A or Never, please explain: (e.g., not met anyone, no interest)

_____

_____

On a scale of 1 to 10, overall how important is it for you to be good in the areas of friendship and social activities just mentioned (solo, meaningful activities, balancing time alone and with others, develop new friendships, spending time with best friends or buddies)?

1 2 3 4 5 6 7 8 9 10
(not at all important)   (extremely important)

Comments:_____

_____

_____

4. Intimacy

4.1 DATING

4.1.A I am quite comfortable dating.

Totally Disagree   Disagree   Agree   Totally Agree

4.1.B In the past 3 months, I have been dating.

Never   Sometimes   Often   Always   N/A
        (had 2 dates or less)   (more than 3 dates)   (have been seeing
                                                          someone weekly)

If N/A or Never, please explain: (e.g., no interest, too trying)

_____

_____

4.2 HAVING BOYFRIEND/GIRLFRIEND OR SPOUSE

4.2.A I enjoy having a stable boy/girlfriend or spouse.

Totally Disagree   Disagree   Agree   Totally Agree

4.2.B In the past 3 months, I have spent time with my stable boy/girlfriend or spouse.

Never   Sometimes   Often   Always   N/A
(every few weeks)   (once a week, for   (weekly for more than
less than a month)   a month)

If N/A or Never, please explain: (e.g., never had a boy/girlfriend, not interested)

_____

_____

4.3 SEXUAL RELATIONSHIP

4.3.A I am interested in sex.

Totally Disagree   Disagree   Agree   Totally Agree

4.3.B In the past 3 months, I have had sex with someone.

Never   Sometimes   Often   Always   N/A
(at least once)   (twice a month or more)   (weekly)

If N/A or Never, please explain: (e.g., religious beliefs, not interested)

_____

_____

4.4 EMOTIONAL CLOSENESS

4.4.A I feel I am able to share feelings, inner thoughts, and be close with my stable boy/girlfriend or spouse (when I have one).

Totally Disagree   Disagree   Agree   Totally Agree

4.4.B In the past 3 months, I have shared my feelings, inner thoughts, and have been close with my stable boy/girlfriend or spouse.

Never   Sometimes   Often   Always   N/A
(at least once)   (twice or more/month)   (weekly or more)

If N/A or Never, please explain: (e.g., no one to share with, not interested)

_____

_____

4.5 Grasping situations

4.5.A I can quickly understand what is going on in most situations involving other people.

Totally Disagree   Disagree   Agree   Totally Agree

4.5.B In the past 3 months, I have been able to quickly understand most situations involving other people.

Never	Sometimes (less than weekly)	Often (most days)	Always (every day)	N/A

If N/A or Never, please explain: (e.g., no need to)

_____

_____

On a scale of 1 to 10, overall how important is it for you to be good in the areas of intimacy just mentioned (dating, having a boy/girlfriend/spouse, sex, emotional closeness, and grasping situations)?

1   2   3   4   5   6   7   8   9   10
(not at all important)   (extremely important)

Comments:_____

_____

_____

5. Family

5.1 Parents

5.1.A I can talk to my parents about things that matter to me.

Totally Disagree   Disagree   Agree   Totally Agree

5.1.B In the past 3 months, I have talked to my parents about things that matter to me.

Never	Sometimes (once a month)	Often (every 2 weeks)	Always (weekly)	N/A

If N/A or Never, please explain: (e.g., don't have contact with parents)

_____

_____

5.2 RELATIONSHIP WITH PARENTS

5.2.A My parents and I typically get along.

Totally Disagree   Disagree   Agree   Totally Agree

5.2.B In the past 3 months, I have spent time without big conflicts with one (or both) of my parents.

Never   Sometimes   Often   Always   N/A
          (less than once/month)   (at least once a month)   (weekly)

If N/A or Never, please explain: (e.g., don't have contact with parents)

_____

_____

5.3 RELATIONSHIP WITH FAMILY

5.3.A I get along well with my family (siblings, grandparents, uncles, aunts, cousins).

Totally Disagree   Disagree   Agree   Totally Agree

5.3.B In the past 3 months, I have spent time (live or phone or other means) with at least one member of my family.

Never   Sometimes   Often   Always   N/A
          (once)   (at least once a month)   (weekly)

If N/A or Never, please explain: (e.g., no extended family, not interested)

_____

_____

On a scale of 1 to 10, how important is it for you to be good in the areas of family just mentioned (being able to talk and not being in conflict with parents, getting along with family)?

          1 2 3 4 5 6 7 8 9 10
(not at all important)   (extremely important)

Comments:_____

_____

_____

6. Relationships and social activities at work (include current and jobs held in the past year)

○ I have not worked in the past year (go to section 8).

6.1 RELATIONSHIP WITH YOUR SUPERVISOR

6.1.A I usually feel comfortable discussing issues related to work with my supervisor (e.g., tasks, feedback, schedules, etc.).

Totally Disagree   Disagree   Agree   Totally Agree

6.1.B In the past 3 months, I have discussed issues related to my job with my supervisor.

| Never | Sometimes (only once when I didn't have a choice) | Often (once or twice by my own initiative) | Always (more than twice by my own initiative) | N/A |

If N/A or Never, please explain: (e.g., have had no problems)

_____

_____

6.2 RELATIONSHIP WITH YOUR CO-WORKERS

6.2.A I typically get along with my co-workers.

Totally Disagree   Disagree   Agree   Totally Agree

6.2.B In the past 3 months, I have spent time with co-workers (talking about work or not).

| Never | Sometimes (once a month) | Often (once a week) | Always (most days) | N/A |

If N/A or Never, please explain: (e.g., no interaction with co-workers, no interest)

_____

_____

6.3 Participation in social activities at work

6.3.A I participate in social activities on the job (Christmas party, after-work outings, etc.).

Totally Disagree   Disagree   Agree   Totally Agree

6.3.B In the past 3 months, I was able to participate in social activities on the job (Christmas party, after-work outings, etc.).

Never	Sometimes (once or twice a year)	Often (once or twice in 6 months)	Always (once or twice in 3 months)	N/A

If N/A or Never, please explain: (e.g., no planned activities, not interested)

_____

_____

On a scale of 1 to 10, overall how important is it for you to be good in the areas of work just mentioned (relationship with supervisor and co-workers, social activities at work)?

          1 2 3 4 5 6 7 8 9 10

(not at all important)   **(extremely important)**

Comments:_____

_____

_____

7. Work abilities (include current and jobs held in the past year)

7.1 Punctuality

7.1.A I always respect my work schedule (get to work on time and leave on time).

Totally Disagree   Disagree   Agree   Totally Agree

7.1.b In the past 3 months, I have respected my work schedule.

Never   Sometimes   Often   Always   N/A
           (once a week)   (once or several times a week)   (each day)

If N/A or Never, please explain: (e.g., set my own schedule)

_____

_____

7.2 Productivity and planning

7.2.a I do my work tasks within the expected time frame.

Totally Disagree   Disagree   Agree   Totally Agree

7.2.b In the past 3 months, I was able to do work tasks within the expected time frame.

Never   Sometimes   Often   Always   N/A
           (once a month)   (once a week)   (several times a week)

If N/A or Never, please explain: (e.g., no tasks with deadlines)

_____

_____

7.3 Quality of work

7.3.a I consistently provide a good quality of work.

Totally Disagree   Disagree   Agree   Totally Agree

7.3.b In the past 3 months, I was able to provide a good quality of work.

Never   Sometimes   Often   Always   N/A
      (once or twice a month)   (once or twice a week)   (every day)

If N/A or Never, please explain: (e.g., job difficulties)

_____

_____

On a scale of 1 to 10, overall how important is it for you to be good in the areas of work just mentioned (punctuality, productivity, and quality of work)?

1 2 3 4 5 6 7 8 9 10

(not at all important)   (extremely important)

Comments:_____

_____

_____

If no job or never worked:

1. Are you looking for work? | Yes | No |

2. Are you enrolled in a vocational program? | Yes | No |

If yes, which one? Name of the program: [   ]

3. Are you in contact with an employment specialist/job coach? | Yes | No |

---

8. School relationships and social activities at school (include current and courses in the past year):

○ I have not attended school (include college, university, or an educational program) in the past year (go to end of document).

8.1 RELATIONSHIP WITH YOUR TEACHER/PROFESSOR

8.1.A I am able to talk to my teacher/professor about things at school/college/ university that matter to me (classes, assignments, schedules, etc.).

Totally Disagree   Disagree   Agree   Totally Agree

8.1.B In the past 3 months, I have talked to my teacher/professor about things at school/college/university that matter to me (classes, assignments, schedules, etc.).

Never   Sometimes   Often   Always   N/A
          (only once when   (once or twice by my (more than twice by
          I didn't have a choice) own initiative)   my own initiative)

If N/A or Never, please explain: (e.g., no problems with classes)

_____

_____

8.2 Relationship with students

8.2.a The other students and I typically get along.

Totally Disagree   Disagree   Agree   Totally Agree

8.2.b In the past 3 months, I have spent time with other students (talking about classes or not).

Never   Sometimes   Often   Always   N/A
             (once a month)   (once a week)   (most days)

If N/A or Never, please explain: (e.g., no interaction with other students)

_____

_____

8.3 Participation in the classroom

8.3.a I am comfortable participating in the classroom.

Totally Disagree   Disagree   Agree   Totally Agree

8.3.b In the past 3 months, I participated in the classroom.

Never   Sometimes   Often   Always   N/A
             (once or twice a   (once or twice   (several times
             month)   a week)   a week)

If N/A or Never, please explain: (e.g., not interested)

_____

_____

On a scale of 1 to 10, overall how important is it for you to be good in the areas of school mentioned (relationship with teachers and students, participation in class)?

1 2 3 4 5 6 7 8 9 10
(not at all important) (extremely important)

Comments:_____

_____

_____

9. Educational abilities

9.1 Meeting deadlines

9.1.A I am always able to finish my assignments on time.

Totally Disagree   Disagree   Agree   Totally Agree

9.1.B In the past 3 months, I was able to hand in assignments on time.

| Never | Sometimes (once or twice) | Often (most of the time) | Always (all of the time) | N/A |

If N/A or Never, please explain: (e.g., arrangements made about assignment deadlines)

_____

_____

9.2 Punctuality

9.2.A I come to the school/college/university on time and rarely miss classes.

Totally Disagree   Disagree   Agree   Totally Agree

9.2.B In the past 3 months, I have been on time for classes and not missed any.

| Never | Sometimes (once a week) | Often (several times a week) | Always (every day) | N/A |

If N/A or Never, please explain: (e.g., no class time)

_____

_____

9.3 Quality of grades

9.3.A I am able to consistently get good grades.

Totally Disagree   Disagree   Agree   Totally Agree

9.3.B In the past 3 months, I have gotten good grades for my assignments and tests/exams.

Never   Sometimes   Often   Always   N/A
    (once or twice)   (most of the time) (all the time)

If N/A or Never, please explain: (e.g., no grading)

_____

_____

On a scale of 1 to 10, overall how important is it for you to be good in the areas of school mentioned (meeting deadlines, punctuality, quality of grades)?

          1 2   3   4   5   6   7   8   9 10
(not at all important)   **(extremely important)**

Comments:_____

_____

_____

If no school or courses:		
1. Are you looking for work?	Yes	No
2. Are you enrolled in an educational program?	Yes	No
If yes, which one? Name of the program:		
3. Are you in contact with a school counsellor?	Yes	No

QuickLL
(Lecomte & Leclerc, 2003)

Client name:_____   Client number_____
Date:_____   Pre-group ☐ or Post-group ☐
                                            (tick: Y)

For each question, circle the answer that you feel is right at this moment. Don't think too much about it and circle what first comes to mind.

1. Right now, your future appears:

not as good   same as usual   better than usual

2. The group therapy is:

making things worse for me   doesn't change anything   making things better for me

3. The group members are:

not nice to me   ok   helpful

4. The group therapists are:

not helpful   ok   helpful and understanding

5. Right now I feel (circle one for each line):

a) nervous   same as usual   calm
b) Sad   same as usual   happy
c) less trustful   same as usual   I can trust people

d) angry	same as usual	peaceful
e) lonely	same as usual	I have one or many friends

6. Right now:

a) I hate myself	I feel the same as usual	I like myself
b) others hate me	others are the same as usual	others like me

7. Right now I have:

a) more voices than usual	same	less voices than usual
b) more distressful thoughts	same	less distressful thoughts than usual

8. Right now:

I feel unable to meet my goals	same	better able to meet my goals

References

CHAPTER 1

Bellack, A. S., Mueser, K. T., Gingerich, S., & Agresta, J. (2004). *Social skills training for schizophrenia: A step-by-step guide* (2nd ed.). New York, NY: Guilford Press.

Bour, P. (1983). The contribution of Jacob Lévy Moreno. *Annales Medico Psychologiques* (Paris), *141*, 1079–1087.

Davidson, L., Chinman, M., Sells, D., & Rowe, M. (2006). Peer support among adults with serious mental illness: A report from the field. *Schizophrenia Bulletin*, *32*, 443–450.

Gabrovsek, V. P. (2009). Inpatient group therapy of patients with schizophrenia. *Psychiatria Danubina*, *21*(Suppl. 1), 67–72.

Kanas, N. (1996). *Group therapy for schizophrenic patients*. Washington, DC: American Psychiatric Press.

Kopelowicz, A., Liberman, R. P., & Zarate, R. (2006). Recent advances in social skills training for schizophrenia. *Schizophrenia Bulletin*, *32*, S12–S23.

Liberman, R. P. (1992). *Handbook of psychiatric rehabilitation* (Vol. 166). University of Michigan Pergamon General Psychology Series.

McGurk, S., Mueser, K. T., & Pascaris, A. (2005). Cognitive training and supported employment for persons with severe mental illness: One year results from a randomized controlled trial. *Schizophrenia Bulletin*, *31*, 898–909.

Moritz, S., Kerstan, A., Veckenstedt, R., Randjbar, S., Vitzthum, F., Schmidt, C., . . . Woodward, T. S. (2011). Further evidence for the efficacy of a metacognitive group training in schizophrenia. *Behaviour Research and Therapy*, *49*, 151–157.

Mueser, K. T., Deavers, F., Penn, D. L., & Cassisi, J. E. (2013). Psychosocial treatments for schizophrenia. *Annual Review of Clinical Psychology*, *9*, 465–497.

Mueser, K. T., Drake, R., & Wallach, M. A. (1998). Dual diagnosis: A review of etiological theories. *Addictive Behaviors*, *23*, 717–734.

Mueser, K. T., Noordsy, D. L., Drake, R. E., & Fox, L. B. (2003). *Integrated treatment for dual disorders: A guide to effective practice*. New York, NY: Guilford Press.

Norcross, J. C., & Wampold, B. E. (2011). Evidence-based therapy relationships: Research conclusions and clinical practices. *Psychotherapy* (Chic), *48*, 98–102.

Prochaska, J. O., DiClemente, C. C., & Norcross, J. C. (1992). In search of how people change: Applications to addictive behaviours. *American Psychologist*, *47*, 1102–1114.

PsychiatricNursing. (2011). Nurses' role in milieu therapy. Retrieved from http://www.nursingplanet.com/pn/milieu_therapy.html

Roder, V., Mueller, D. R., Mueser, K. T., & Brenner, H. D. (2006). Integrated psychological therapy (IPT) for schizophrenia: Is it effective? *Schizophrenia Bulletin, 32*(Suppl. 1), S81–S93.

Ruddy, R. A., & Dent-Brown, K. (2007, January 24). Drama therapy for schizophrenia or schizophrenia-like illnesses. *Cochrane Database Systematic Review.*

Townsend, M. C., Clavet, H., Desbiens, R., Robitaille, I., Benoit, A., Leclerc, C., . . . Genest, C. (2010). *Soins infirmiers: Psychiatrie et santé mentale.* Montreal: Édition du Renouveau Pédagogique.

Wykes, T., Parr, A.-M., & Landau, S. (1999). Group treatment of auditory hallucinations. *British Journal of Psychiatry, 175,* 180–185.

Yalom, I. D. (1983). *Inpatient group psychotherapy.* New York, NY: Basic Books.

Yalom, I. D., & Leszcz, M. (2005*). The theory and practice of group psychotherapy* (5th ed.). New York, NY: Basic Books.

Yalom, I. D., & Lieberman, M. A. (1971). A study of encounter group casualties. *Archives of General Psychiatry, 25,* 16–30.

CHAPTER 2

Andresen, R., Oades, L., & Caputi, P. (2003). The experience of recovery from schizophrenia: Towards an empirically validated stage model. *Australian and New Zealand Journal of Psychiatry, 37,* 586–594. doi:1234 [pii]

Anselmetti, S., Cavallaro, R., Bechi, M., Angelone, S. M., Ermoli, E., Cocchi, F., & Smeraldi, E. (2007). Psychopathological and neuropsychological correlates of source monitoring impairment in schizophrenia. *Psychiatry Research, 150,* 51–59.

Arseneault, L., Cannon, M., Fisher, H. L., Polanczyk, G., Moffitt, T. E., & Caspi, A. (2011). Childhood trauma and children's emerging psychotic symptoms: A genetically sensitive longitudinal cohort study. *American Journal of Psychiatry, 168,* 65–72. doi:10.1176/appi.ajp.2010.10040567

Bandura, A. (1977). *Social learning theory.* New York, NY: General Learning Press.

Beck, A. T., & Rector, N. A. (2005). Cognitive approaches to schizophrenia: Theory and therapy. *Annual Review of Clinical Psychology, 1,* 577–606. doi:0.1146/annurev.clinpsy.1.102803.144205

Beck, A. T., Rush, A. J., Shaw, B. F., & Emery, G. (1979). *Cognitive therapy of depression.* New York, NY: Guilford Press.

Bentall, R. P., & Slade, P. D. (1985). Reality testing and auditory hallucinations: A signal-detection analysis. *British Journal of Clinical Psychology, 24,* 159–169.

Bentall, R. P., Wickham, S., Shevlin, M., & Varese, F. (2012). Do specific early-life adversities lead to specific symptoms of psychosis? A study from the 2007 Adult Psychiatric Morbidity Survey. *Schizophrenia Bulletin, 38,* 734–740. doi:10.1093/schbul/sbs049

Berrios, G. (1991). Delusions as "wrong beliefs": A conceptual history. *British Journal of Psychiatry, 159,* 6–13.

Birchwood, M., Meaden, A., Trower, P., Gilbert, P., & Plaistow, J. (2000). The power and omnipotence of voices: Subordination and entrapment by voices and significant others. *Psychological Medicine, 30,* 337–344.

Bonoldi, I., Simeone, E., Rocchetti, M., Codjoe, L., Rossi, G., Gambi, F., . . . Fusar-Poli, P. (2013). Prevalence of self-reported childhood abuse in psychosis: A meta-analysis of retrospective studies. *Psychiatry Research, 30,* 8–15. doi:10.1016/j.psychres.2013.05.003

Brett-Jones, J., Garety, P., & Hemsley, D. (1987). Measuring delusional experiences: A method and its application. *British Journal of Clinical Psychology, 26,* 257–265.

El-Khoury, B., & Lecomte, T. (2012). Emotional regulation and schizophrenia. *International Journal of Cognitive Therapy, 51,* 67–76.

Garety, P. A., Hemsley, D. R., & Wessely, S. (1991). Reasoning in deluded schizophrenic and paranoid patients: Biases in performance on a probabilistic inference task. *Journal of Nervous and Mental Disease, 179,* 194–201.

Hemsley, D. R. (1996). Schizophrenia: A cognitive model and its implication for psychological intervention. *Behavior Modification, 20,* 139–169.

Hoffman, R. E. (1986). Verbal hallucinations and language production processes in schizophrenia. *Behavioral and Brain Sciences, 9,* 503–548.

Kinderman, P., & Bentall, R. P. (2000). Self-discrepancies and causal attributions: Studies of hypothesized relationships. *British Journal of Clinical Psychology, 39*, 255–273.

Kingdon, D., Turkington, D., & John, C. (1994). Cognitive behaviour therapy of schizophrenia. The amenability of delusions and hallucinations to reasoning. *British Journal of Psychiatry, 164*, 581–587.

Liberman, R. P. (1982). What is schizophrenia? *Schizophrenia Bulletin, 8*, 435–437.

Liberman, R. P., & Kopelowicz, A. (2005). Recovery from schizophrenia: A concept in search of research. *Psychiatric Services, 56*, 735–742. doi:56/6/735 [pii] 10.1176/appi.ps.56.6.735

Lysaker, P. H., Gumley, A., Luedtke, B., Buck, K. D., Ringer, J. M., Olesek, K., ... Dimaggio, G. (2013). Social cognition and metacognition in schizophrenia: Evidence of their independence and linkage with outcomes. *Acta Psychiatrica Scandinavica, 127*, 239–247. doi:10.1111/acps.12012

Lysaker, P. H., & Salyers, M. P. (2007). Anxiety symptoms in schizophrenia spectrum disorders: Associations with social function, positive and negative symptoms, hope and trauma history. *Acta Psychiatrica Scandinavica, 116*, 290–298.

Mueser, K. T., Rosenberg, S. D., Goodman, L. A., & Trumbetta, S. L. (2002). Trauma, PTSD, and the course of severe mental illness: An interactive model. *Schizophrenia Research, 53*, 123–143.

Mueser, K. T., Yarnold, P. R., Levinson, D. F., Singh, H., Bellack, A. S., Kee, K., ... Yadalam, K. G. (1990). Prevalence of substance abuse in schizophrenia: Demographic and clinical correlates. *Schizophrenia Bulletin, 16*, 31–56.

Noiseux, S., St-Cyr Tribble, D., Leclerc, C., Ricard, N., Corin, E., Morissette, R., & Lambert, R. (2009). Developing a model of recovery in mental health. *BMC Health Services Research, 9*, 73. doi:10.1186/1472-6963-9-73

Noordsy, D. L., Torrey, W. C., Mueser, K. T., Mead, S., O'Keefe, C., & Fox, L. (2002). Recovery from severe mental illness: An intrapersonal and functional outcome definition. *International Review of Psychiatry, 14*, 318–326.

Salvatore, G., Dimaggio, G., Popolo, R., & Lysaker, P. H. (2008). Deficits in mindreading in stressful contexts and their relationships to social withdrawal in schizophrenia. *Bulletin of the Menninger Clinic, 72*, 191–209.

Semmelhack, D., Ende, L., & Hazell, C. (2013). *Group therapy for adults with severe mental illness: Adapting the Tavistock method*. New York, NY: Routledge.

Shepherd, G., Boardman, J., & Slade, M. (2008). *Making recovery a reality. Sainsbury Center for Mental Health*. London, UK.

Silverstein, S. M., & Bellack, A. S. (2008). A scientific agenda for the concept of recovery as it applies to schizophrenia. *Clinincal Psycholology Review, 28*, 1108–1124. doi:10.1016/j.cpr.2008.03.004

Stephane, M., Barton, S., & Boutros, N. N. (2001). Auditory verbal hallucinations and dysfunction of the neural substrates of speech. *Schizophrenia Research, 50*, 61–78.

Udachina, A., Varese, F., Oorschot, M., Myin-Germeys, I., & Bentall, R. P. (2013). Dynamics of self-esteem in "poor-me" and "bad-me" paranoia. *Journal of Nervous and Mental Disease, 200*, 777–783. doi:10.1097/NMD.0b013e318266ba57

Varese, F., Smeets, F., Drukker, M., Lieverse, R., Lataster, T., Viechtbauer, W., ... Bentall, R. P. (2012). Childhood adversities increase the risk of psychosis: A meta-analysis of patient-control, prospective- and cross-sectional cohort studies. *Schizophrenia Bulletin, 38*, 661–671. doi:10.1093/schbul/sbs050

Walen, S. R., DiGiuseppe, R., & Dryden, W. (1992). A practitioner's guide to rational-emotive therapy (2nd ed.).

Wickett, A., Essman, W., Beck-Jennings, J., Davis, L., McIlvried, J., & Lysaker, P. H. (2006). Cluster B and C personality traits, symptom correlates, and treatment utilization in postacute schizophrenia. *Journal of Nervous and Mental Disease, 194*, 650–653.

Wigman, J. T., van Nierop, M., Vollebergh, W. A., Lieb, R., Beesdo-Baum, K., Wittchen, H. U., & van Os, J. (2012). Evidence that psychotic symptoms are prevalent in disorders of anxiety and depression, impacting on illness onset, risk, and severity: Implications for diagnosis and ultra-high risk research. *Schizophrenia Bulletin, 38*, 247–257.

Woodward, T. S., Munz, M., Leclerc, C., & Lecomte, T. (2009). Change in delusions is associated with change in "jumping to conclusions." *Psychiatry Research, 170*, 124–127. doi:S0165-1781(08)00388-0 [pii] 10.1016/j.psychres.2008.10.020

Young, J. E., Klosko, J. S., & Weishaar, M. E. (2003). *Schema therapy: A practitioner's guide*. New York, NY: Guilford Press.

Zubin, J., & Spring, B. (1977). Vulnerability: A new view on schizophrenia. *Journal of Abnormal Psychology*, *86*, 103–126.

CHAPTER 3

Addington, J., Epstein, I., Liu, L., French, P., Boydell, K. M., & Zipursky, R. B. (2011). A randomized controlled trial of cognitive behavioral therapy for individuals at clinical high risk of psychosis. *Schizophrenia Research*, *125*, 54–61. doi:10.1016/j.schres.2010.10.015

Allott, K., Alvarez-Jimenez, M., Killackey, E. J., Bendall, S., McGorry, P. D., & Jackson, H. J. (2011). Patient predictors of symptom and functional outcome following cognitive behaviour therapy or befriending in first-episode psychosis. *Schizophrenia Research*, *132*, 125–130.

Álvarez-Jiménez, M., Parker, A. G., Hetrick, S. E., McGorry, P. D., & Gleeson, J. F. (2011). Preventing the second episode: A systematic review and meta-analysis of psychosocial and pharmacological trials in first-episode psychosis. *Schizophrenia Bulletin*, *37*, 619–630.

Barrowclough, C., Haddock, G., Lobban, F., Jones, S., Siddle, R., Roberts, C., & Gregg, L. (2006). Group cognitive–behavioural therapy for schizophrenia Randomised controlled trial. *The British Journal of Psychiatry*, *189*(6), 527–532; doi:10.1192/bjp.bp.106.021386

Beauchamp, M-C., Lecomte, T., Lecomte, C., Leclerc, C., & Corbière, M. (2013). Do personality traits matter when choosing a group therapy for early psychosis? *Psychology and Psychotherapy: Theory, Research and Practice*, *86*(1), 19–32.

Bentall, R., Tarrier, N., Lewis, S., Haddock, G., Kinderman, P., Kingdon, D., & the SoCRATES team. (2002). The therapeutic alliance in early psychosis. *Acta Psychiatrica Scandinavica*, *106*(s413), 69–106.

Berry, C., & Hayward, M. (2011). What can qualitative research tell us about service user perspectives of CBT for psychosis? A synthesis of current evidence. *Behavioural and Cognitive Psychotherapy*, *39*, 487–494.

Birchwood, M., Peters, E., Tarrier, N., Dunn, G., Lewis, S., Wykes, T., . . . Michail, M. (2011). A multi-centre, randomised controlled trial of cognitive therapy to prevent harmful compliance with command hallucinations. *BMC Psychiatry*, *11*(155). doi:10.1186/1471-244X-11-155

Birchwood, M., & Trower, P. (2006). The future of cognitive-behavioural therapy for psychosis: Not a quasi-neuroleptic. *British Journal of Psychiatry*, *188*, 107–108.

Borras, L., Boucherie, M., Mohr, S., Lecomte, T., Perroud, N., & Huguelet, P. (2009). Increasing self-esteem: efficacy of a group intervention for individuals with severe mental disorders. *Eur Psychiatry*, *24*(5), 307–316. doi:10.1016/j.eurpsy.2009.01.003

Brabban, A., Tai, S., & Turkington, D. (2009). Predictors of outcome in brief cognitive behavior therapy for schizophrenia. *Schizophrenia Bulletin*, *35*, 859–864.

Burns, A. M. N., Erickson, D. H., Brenner, C. A. (2014). Cognitive-behavior therapy for medication-resistant psychosis: A meta-analytic review. *Psychiatric Services*, *65*, 874–880.

Chadwick, P., Hughes, S., Russell, D., Russell, I., & Dagnan, D. (2009). Mindfulness groups for distressing voices and paranoia: A replication and randomized feasibility trial. *Behavioural and Cognitive Psychotherapy*, *37*, 403–412. doi:10.1017/S1352465809990166

Chadwick, P. D., & Lowe, C. F. (1990). Measurement and modification of delusional beliefs. *Journal of Consulting and Clinical Psychology*, *58*, 225–232.

Dixon, L. B., Dickerson, F., Bellack, A. S., Bennett, M., Dickinson, D., Goldberg, R. W., . . . Kreyenbuhl, J. (2010). Schizophrenia Patient Outcomes Research Team (PORT): The 2009 schizophrenia PORT: Psychosocial treatment recommendations and summary statements. *Schizophrenia Bulletin*, *36*, 48–70.

Drury, V., Birchwood, M., Cochrane, R., & Macmillan, F. (1996). Cognitive therapy and recovery from acute psychosis: A controlled trial. *British Journal of Psychiatry*, *169*, 593–601.

Dunn, G., Fowler, D., Rollinson, R., Garety, P., Freeman, D., Kuipers, E., . . . Garety, P. (2012). Effective elements of CBT for psychosis. *Psychological Medicine*, *42*, 1057–1068.

Dunn, H., Morrison, A. P., & Bentall, R. P. (2006). The relationship between patient suitability, therapeutic alliance, homework compliance and outcome in cognitive therapy for psychosis. *Clinical Psychology and Psychotherapy, 13*, 145–152.

Durham, R. C., Guthrie, M., Morton, R. V., Reid, D. A., Treliving, L. R., Fowler, D., & Macdonald, R. R. (2003). Tayside-Fife clinical trial of cognitive-behavioural therapy for medication-resistant psychotic symptoms: Results to 3-month follow-up. *British Journal of Psychiatry, 182*, 303–311.

Flach, C., French, P., Dunn, G., Fowler, D., Gumley, A. I., Birchwood, M., . . . Morrison, A. P. (2015). Components of therapy as mechanisms of change in cognitive therapy for people at risk of psychosis: Analysis of the EDIE-2 trial. *British Journal of Psychiatry, 1*, 7. doi:10.1192/bjp.bp.114.153320

Freeman, D., Dunn, G., Garety, P., Weinman, J., Kuipers, E., Fowler, D., . . . Bebbington, P. (2013). Patients' beliefs about the causes, persistence and control of psychotic experiences predict take-up of effective cognitive behaviour therapy for psychosis. *Psychological Medicine, 43*, 269–277.

Freeman, D., Dunn, G., Startup, H., & Kingdon, D. (2015). An explanatory randomised controlled trial testing the effects of targeting worry in patients with persistent persecutory delusions: The Worry Intervention Trial (WIT). *Efficacy and Mechanism Evaluation, 2*, 1–36. doi:10.3310/eme02010

Garety, P., Fowler, D., Kuipers, E., Freeman, D., Dunn, G., Bebbington, P., . . . Jones, S. (1997). London–East Anglia randomised controlled trial of cognitive-behaviour therapy for psychosis. II. Predictors of outcome. *British Journal of Psychiatry, 171*, 420–426.

Gleeson, J. F., Cotton, S. M., Alvarez-Jimenez, M., Wade, D., Gee, D., Crisp, K., . . . McGorry, P. D. (2013). A randomized controlled trial of relapse prevention therapy for first-episode psychosis patients: Outcome at 30-month follow-up. *Schizophrenia Bulletin, 39*, 436–448. doi:10.1093/schbul/sbr165

Gottlieb, J. D., Romeo, K. H., Penn, D. L., Mueser, K. T., & Chiko, B. P. (2013). Web-based cognitive-behavioral therapy for auditory hallucinations in persons with psychosis: A pilot study. *Schizophrenia Research, 145*, 82–87. doi:10.1016/j.schres.2013.01.002

Gould, R. A., Mueser, K. T., Bolton, E., Mays, V., & Goff, D. (2001). Cognitive therapy for psychosis in schizophrenia: An effect size analysis. *Schizophrenia Research, 48*, 335–342.

Granholm, E., Ben-Zeev, D., & Link, P. C. (2009). Social disinterest attitudes and group cognitive-behavioral social skills training for functional disability in schizophrenia. *Schizophrenia Bulletin, 35*, 874–883. doi:10.1093/schbul/sbp072

Granholm, E., McQuaid, J. R., McClure, F. S., Auslander, L. A., Perivoliotis, D., Pedrelli, P., . . . Jeste, D.V. (2005). A randomized, controlled trial of cognitive behavioral social skills training for middle-aged and older outpatients with chronic schizophrenia. *American Journal of Psychiatry, 162*, 520–529.

Grant, P. M., Huh, G. A., Perivoliotis, D., Stolar, N. M., & Beck, A. T. (2012). Randomized trial to evaluate the efficacy of cognitive therapy for low-functioning patients with schizophrenia. *Archives of General Psychiatry, 69*, 121–127. doi:10.1001/archgenpsychiatry.2011.129

Gumley, A., O'Grady, M., McNay, L., Reilly, J., Power, K., & Norrie, J. (2003). Early intervention for relapse in schizophrenia: Results of a 12-month randomized controlled trial of cognitive behavioural therapy. *Psychological Medicine, 33*, 419–431.

Hofmann, S. G., Asnaani, A., Vonk, I. J. J., Sawyer, A. T., & Fang, A. (2012). The efficacy of cognitive behavioral therapy: A review of meta-analyses. *Cognitive Therapy and Research, 36*, 427–440.

Hutton, P., & Taylor, P. J. (2013). Cognitive behavioural therapy for psychosis prevention: A systematic review and meta-analysis. *Psychological Medicine, 22*, 1–20.

Jackson, H., McGorry, P., Henry, L., Edwards, J., Hulbert, C., Harrigan, S., . . . Power, P. (2001). Cognitively oriented psychotherapy for early psychosis (COPE): A 1-year follow-up. *British Journal of Clinical Psychology, 40*, 57–70.

Jauhar, S., McKenna, P. J., Radua, J., Fung, E., Salvador, R., & Laws, K. R. (2014). Cognitive-behavioural therapy for the symptoms of schizophrenia: Systematic review and meta-analysis with examination of potential bias. *British Journal of Psychiatry, 204*, 20–29. doi:10.1192/bjp.bp.112.116285

Johnson, D. P., Penn, D. L., Bauer, D. J., Meyer, P., & Evans, E. (2008). Predictors of the therapeutic alliance in group therapy for individuals with treatment-resistant auditory hallucinations. *British Journal of Clinical Psychology, 47*, 171–183.

Joyce, A. S., Piper, W. E., & Ogrodniczuk, J. S. (2007). Therapeutic alliance and cohesion variables as predictors of outcome in short-term group psychotherapy. *International Journal of Group Psychotherapy, 57*, 269–296.

Klingberg, S., Wölwer, W., Engel, C., Wittorf, A., Herrlich, J., Meisner, C., . . . Wiedemann, G. (2011). Negative symptoms of schizophrenia as primary target of cognitive behavioral therapy: Results of the randomized clinical TONES study. *Schizophrenia Bulletin, 37*(Suppl. 2), S98–S110. doi:10.1093/schbul/sbr073

Kråkvik, B., Gråwe, R. W., Hagen, R., & Stiles, T. C. (2013). Cognitive behaviour therapy for psychotic symptoms: A randomized controlled effectiveness trial. *Behavioural and Cognitive Psychotherapy, 41*, 511–524.

Kuipers, E., Garety, P., Fowler, D., Freeman, D., Dunn, G., Bebbington, P., & Hadley, C. (1997). London–East Anglia randomised controlled trial of cognitive-behavioural therapy for psychosis: Effects of treatment phase. *British Journal of Psychiatry, 171*, 319–327.

Leclerc, C., & Lecomte, T. (2012). TCC pour premiers épisodes de psychose: Pourquoi la thérapie de groupe obtient les meilleurs résultats? *Journal de Thérapie Comportementale et Cognitive, 22*, 104–110.

Leclerc, C., Lesage, A. D., Ricard, N., Lecomte, T., & Cyr, M. (2000). Assessment of a new stress management module for persons with schizophrenia. *American Journal of Orthopsychiatry, 3*, 380–388.

Lecomte, T., Cyr, M., Lesage, A. D., Wilde, J. B., Leclerc, C., & Ricard, N. (1999). Efficacy of a self-esteem module in the empowerment of individuals with chronic schizophrenia. *Journal of Nervous and Mental Diseases, 187*, 406–413.

Lecomte, T., Laferriere-Simarc, M-C., & Leclerc, C. (2011). What does the alliance predict in group interventions for early psychosis? *Journal of Contemporary Psychotherapy, 42*(2), 55–61.

Lecomte, T., Leclerc, C., Corbière, C., Wykes, T., Wallace, C. J., & Spidel, A. (2008). Group cognitive behaviour therapy or social skills training for individuals with a first episode of psychosis? Results of a randomized controlled trial. *Journal of Nervous and Mental Disease, 196*, 866–875.

Lecomte, T., Leclerc, C., & Wykes, T. (2012). Group CBT for early psychosis: Are there still benefits one year later? *International Journal of Group Psychotherapy, 62*, 309–321.

Lecomte, T., Leclerc, C., Wykes, T., & Lecomte, J. (2003). Group CBT for clients with a first episode of psychosis. *Journal of Cognitive Psychotherapy: An International Quarterly, 17*, 375–384.

Lecomte, T., Corbière, M., & Lysaker, P. (2014). A group cognitive-behaviour therapy for people registered in supported employment programs: CBT-SE. *Encéphale, 40*(Suppl 2), S81–S90. doi:10.1016/j.encep.2014.04.005

Lecomte, T., Leclerc, C., Wykes, T., Nicole, L., & Baki, A. A. (2014), Understanding process in group cognitive behavior therapy for psychosis. *Psychology and Psychotherapy: Theory, Research and Practice.* Advance online publication. doi:10.1111/papt.12039

Leucht, S., Cipriani, A., Spineli, L., Mavridis, D., Örey, D., Richter, F., . . . Davis, J. M. (2013). Comparative efficacy and tolerability of 15 antipsychotic drugs in schizophrenia: A multiple-treatments meta-analysis. *Lancet, 382*, 951–962.

Lewis, S., Tarrier, N., Haddock, G., Bentall, R., Kinderman, P., Kingdon, D., . . . Dunn, G. (2002). Randomized controlled trial of cognitive behavioural therapy in early schizophrenia: Acute-phase outcomes. *British Journal of Psychiatry, 181*(Suppl. 43), S91–S97.

Lynch, D., Laws, K. R., & McKenna, P. J. (2010). Cognitive behavioural therapy for major psychiatric disorder: Does it really work? A meta-analytical review of well-controlled trials. *Psychological Medicine, 40*, 9–24.

Lysaker, P. H., & Roe, D. (2012). The processes of recovery from schizophrenia: The emergent role of integrative psychotherapy, recent developments and new directions. *Journal of Psychotherapy Integration, 22*, 287–297.

Morrison, A. P., & Barratt, S. (2010). What are the components of CBT for psychosis? A Delphi study. *Schizophrenia Bulletin, 36*, 136–142.

Morrison, A. P., French, P., Stewart, S. L., Birchwood, M., Fowler, D., Gumley, A. I., . . . Dunn, G. (2012). Early detection and intervention evaluation for people at risk of psychosis: Multisite randomised controlled trial. *British Medical Journal, 344*(e2233). doi:10.1136/bmj.e2233

Morrison, A. P., Turkington, D., Pyle, M., Spencer, H., Brabban, A., Dunn, G., . . . Hutton, P. (2014). Cognitive therapy for people with schizophrenia spectrum disorders not taking antipsychotic drugs: A single-blind randomised controlled trial. *Lancet, 383*, 1395–1403.

Morrison, A. P., French, P., Walford, L., Lewis, S. W., Kilcommons, A., Green, J., . . . Bentall, R. P. (2004). Cognitive therapy for the prevention of psychosis in people at ultra-high risk: Randomised controlled trial. *British Journal of Psychiatry, 185*, 291–297.

Myhr, G., Russel, J. J., Saint-Laurent, M., Tagalakis, V., Belisle, D., Khodari, F., . . . Pinard, G. (2013). Assessing suitability for short-term cognitive-behavioral therapy in psychiatric outpatients with psychosis: A comparison with depressed and anxious outpatients. *Journal of Psychiatric Practice, 19*(1), 29–41.

Naeem, F., Kingdon, D., & Turkington, D. (2008). Predictors of response to cognitive behavior therapy in the treatment of schizophrenia: A comparison of brief and standard interventions. *Cognitive Therapy Research, 32*, 651–656.

Naeem, F., Saeed, S., Irfan, M., Kiran, T., Mehmood, N., Gul, M., . . . Kingdon, D. (2015). Brief culturally adapted CBT for psychosis (CaCBTp): A randomized controlled trial from a low income country. *Schizophrenia Research, 164*, 143–148.

NICE. (2009). Schizophrenia: Core interventions in the treatment and management of schizophrenia in adults in primary and secondary care (update). National Institute for Health and Care Excellence, U.K.

Ogrodniczuk, J. S., Joyce, A. S., & Piper, W. E. (2003). Changes in perceived social support after group therapy for complicated grief. *Journal of Nervous and Mental Disease, 191*Owen, M., Sellwood, W., Kan, S., Murray, J., & Sarsam, M. (2015). Group CBT for psychosis: A longitudinal, controlled trial with inpatients. *Behaviour Research and Therapy, 65*, 76–85.

Penn, D. L., Meyer, P. S., Evans, E., Wirth, R. J., Cai, K., & Burchinal, M. (2009). A randomized controlled trial of group cognitive-behavioral therapy vs. enhanced supportive therapy for auditory hallucinations. *Schizophrenia Research, 109*(1–3), 52–59. doi:10.1016/j.schres.2008.12.009

Pilling, S., Bebbington, P., Kuipers, E., Garety, P., Geddes, J., Orbach, G., & Morgan, C. (2002). Psychological treatments in schizophrenia: I. Meta-analysis of family intervention and cognitive behaviour therapy. *Psychological Medicine, 32*, 763–782.

Raune, D., & Law, S. (2013). Pilot programme of modular symptom-specific group cognitive behaviour therapy in a 'Real World' early intervention in psychosis service. *Early Intervention Psychiatry, 7*(2), 221–229. doi:10.1111/eip.12025. Epub 2013 Jan 24.

Saksa, J. R., Cohen, S. J., Srihari, V. H., & Woods, S. W. (2009). Cognitive behavior therapy for early psychosis: A comprehensive review of individual vs group treatment studies. *International Journal of Group Psychotherapy, 59*, 357–383.

Sarin, F., Wallin, L., & Widerlöv, B. (2011). Cognitive behavior therapy for schizophrenia: A meta-analytical review of randomized controlled trials. *Nordic Journal of Psychiatry, 65*, 162–174.

Sensky, T., Turkington, D., Kingdon, D., Scott, J. L., Siddle, R., O'Carroll, M., & Barnes, T. R. E. (2000). A randomized controlled trial of cognitive-behavioral therapy for persistent symptoms in schizophrenia resistant to medication. *Archives of General Psychiatry, 57*, 165–172.

Staring, A. B., Ter Huurne, M. A., & van der Gaag, M. (2013). Cognitive behavioral therapy for negative symptoms (CBT-n) in psychotic disorders: A pilot study. *Journal of Behavioural Therapy and Experimental Psychiatry, 44*, 300–306. doi:10.1016/j.jbtep.2013.01.004

Tarrier, N., Beckett, R., Harwood, S., Baker, A., Yusupoff, L., & Ugarteburu, I. (1993). A trial of two cognitive-behavioural methods of treating drug-resistant psychotic symptoms in schizophrenic clients: 1. Outcome. *British Journal of Psychiatry, 162*, 524–532.

Tarrier, N., Yusupoff, L., Kinney, C., MacCarthy, E., Gledhill, A., Haddock, H., & Morris, J. (1998). Randomised controlled trial of intensive cognitive behaviour therapy for chronic schizophrenia. *British Medical Journal, 317*, 303–307.

Thomas, N., Rossell, S., Farhall, J., Shawyer, F., & Castle, D. (2011). Cognitive behavioural therapy for auditory hallucinations: Effectiveness and predictors of outcome in a specialist clinic. *Behavioural and Cognitive Psychotherapy, 39*, 129–138. doi:10.1017/S1352465810000548

Trower, P., Birchwood, M., Meaden, A., Byrne, S., Nelson, A., & Ross, K. (2004). Cognitive therapy for command hallucinations: Randomised controlled trial. *British Journal of Psychiatry, 184*, 312–320.

Turner, D. T., van der Gaag, M., Kariotaki, E., & Cuijpers, P. (2014). Psychological interventions for psychosis: A meta-analysis of comparative outcome studies. *American Journal of Psychiatry, 171*, 523–538.

van der Gaag, M., van Oosterhout, B., Daalman, K., Sommer, I. E., & Korrelboom, K. (2012). Initial evaluation of the effects of competitive memory training (COMET) on depression in schizophrenia-spectrum patients with persistent auditory verbal hallucinations: A randomized controlled trial. *British Journal of Clinical Psychology, 51*, 158–171. doi:10.1111/j.2044-8260.2011.02025.x

Wampold, B., Mondin, G., Moody, M., Stich, F., Benson, K., & Ahn, H. (1997). Methodological problems in identifying efficacious psychotherapies. *Psychotherapy Research, 7*, 21–43.

Wykes, T., Hayward, P., Thomas, N., Green, N., Surguladze, S., Fannon, D., & Landau, S. (2005). What are the effects of group cognitive behaviour therapy for voices? A randomised control trial. *Schizophrenia Research, 77*, 201–210.

Wykes, T., Parr, A-M., & Landau, S. (1999). Group treatment of auditory hallucinations. *British Journal of Psychiatry, 175*, 180–185.

Wykes, T., Steel, C., Everitt, B., & Tarrier, N. (2008). Cognitive behavior therapy for schizophrenia: Effect sizes, clinical models, and methodological rigor. *Schizophrenia Bulletin, 34*, 523–537.

Young, J., & Beck, A. (1980). *The Cognitive Therapy Scale rating manual*. Philadelphia, PA: Beck Institute.

Zimmermann, G., Favrod, J., Trieu, V. H., & Pomini, V. (2005). The effect of cognitive behavioral treatment on the positive symptoms of schizophrenia spectrum disorders: A meta-analysis. *Schizophrenia Research, 77*, 1–9.

CHAPTER 4

Castonguay, L. G., Constantino, M. J., & Holtforth, M. G. (2006). The working alliance: Where are we and where should we go? *Psychotherapy: Theory, Research, Practice, Training, 43*, 271–279.

Lecomte, T., Leclerc, C., Wykes, T., Nicole, L., & Abdel Baki, A. (2015). Understanding process in group cognitive behavior therapy for psychosis. *Psychology and Psychotherapy: Theory, Research and Practice, 88*, 163–177. doi:10.1111/papt.12039.

Lecomte, T., Leclerc, C., & Wykes, T. (2012). Group CBT for early psychosis: Are there still benefits one year later? *International Journal of Group Psychotherapy, 62*, 309–321.

Lecomte, T., Leclerc, C., Corbière, M., Wykes, T., Wallace, C. J., & Spidel, A. (2008). Group cognitive behavior therapy or social skills training for individuals with recent onset of psychosis? Results of a randomized controlled trial. *Journal of Nervous and Mental Disease, 196*, 866–875.

Yalom, I. D., & Leszcz, M. (2005). *The theory and practice of group psychotherapy* (5th ed.). New York, NY: Basic Books.

CHAPTER 5

Liberman, R. P. (1992). *Handbook of psychiatric rehabilitation* (Vol. 166). University of Michigan Pergamon General Psychology Series.

Semmelhack, D., Ende, L., & Hazell, C. (2013). *Group therapy for adults with severe mental illness: Adapting the Tavistock method*. New York, NY: Routledge.

CHAPTER 8

Seligman, M. (2006). *Learned optimism: How to change your mind and your life* (3rd ed.). New York, NY: Random House.

CHAPTER 9

Palmer, B. A., Pankratz, S., & Bostwick, J. M. (2005). The lifetime risk of suicide in schizophrenia: A reexamination. *Archives of General Psychiatry, 62*, 247–253. doi:10.1001/archpsyc.62.3.247

CHAPTER 11

APA. (1987). *Diagnostic and statistical manual of mental disorders* (3rd ed.). Washington, DC.

APA. (1994). *Diagnostic and statistical manual of mental disorders* (4th ed.). Washington, DC.

Birchwood, M., Smith, J., Cochrane, R., & Wetton, S. (1990). The Social Functioning Scale: The development and validation of a new scale of social adjustment for use in family intervention programmes with schizophrenic patients. *British Journal of Psychiatry, 157*, 853–859.

Boyd, J. E., Emerald, P. A., Otilingam, P. G., & Peters, T. (2014). Internalized Stigma of Mental Illness (ISMI) scale: A multinational review. *Comprehensive Psychiatry, 55*, 221–231.

Burlingame, G. M., McClendon, D. T., & Alonso, J. (2011). Cohesion in group therapy. *Psychotherapy (Chic), 48*, 34–42.

Carver, C. S. (1997). You want to measure coping but your protocol's too long: Consider the Brief COPE. *International Journal of Behavioral Medicine, 4*, 92–100.

Carver, C. S., Scheier, M. F., & Weintraub, J. K. (1989). Assessing coping strategies: A theoretically based approach. *Journal of Personality and Social Psychology, 56*, 267–283.

Chapman, C. L., Baker, E. L., Porter, G., Thayer, S. D., & Burlingame, G. M. (2010). Rating group therapist interventions: Validation of the Group Psychotherapy Intervention Rating Scale. *Group Dynamics: Theory, Research and Practice, 14*, 15–31.

Cutrona, C. E., & Russell, D. W. (1987). The provisions of social relationships and adaptation to stress. *Advances in personal relationships,1*, 37–67.

Derogatis, L., & Melisaratos, N. (1983). The Brief Symptom Inventory: An introductory report. *Psychological Medicine, 13*, 595–605.

Drake, R., Haddock, G., Tarrier, N., Bentall, R., & Lewis, S. (2007). The Psychotic Symptom Rating Scales (PSYRATS): Their usefulness and properties in first episode psychosis. *Schizophrenia Research, 89*, 119–122.

Edwards, J. R., & Baglioni, A. J., Jr. (1993). The measurement of coping with stress: Construct validity of the Ways of Coping Checklist and the Cybernetic Coping Scale. *Work & Stress, 7*, 17–31.

Endler, N. S., & Parker, J. D. A. (1990). *Coping Inventory for Stressful Situations (CISS): Manual.* Toronto, Ontario, Canada: Multi-Health Systems.

Gottlieb, B. H., & Bergen, A. E. (2010). Social support concepts and measures. *Journal of Psychosomatic Research, 69*, 511–520.

Greenwood, K. E., Sweeney, A., Williams, S., Garety, P., Kuipers, E., Scott, J., & Peters, E. (2010). CHoice of Outcome In Cbt for psychosEs (CHOICE): The development of a new service-user led outcome measure of CBT for psychosis. *Schizophrenia Bulletin, 36*, 126–135.

Guppy, A., Edwards, J. A., Brough, P., Peters-Bean, K. M., Sale, C., & Short, E. (2004). The psychometric properties of the short version of the Cybernetic Coping Scale: A multigroup confirmatory factor analysis across four samples. *Journal of Occupational and Organizational Psychology, 77*, 39–62.

Haddock, G., Devane, S., Bradshaw, T., McGovern, J., Tarrier, N., Kinderman, P., . . . Harris, N. (2001). An investigation into the psychometric properties of the Cognitive Therapy Scale for Psychosis (CTS-Psy). *Behavioural and Cognitive Psychotherapy, 29*, 221–233.

Hatcher, R. L., & Gillaspy, J. A. (2006). Development and validation of a revised short version of the Working Alliance Inventory. *Psychotherapy Research, 16*, 12–25.

Horvath, A. O., & Greenberg, L. S. (1989). Development and validation of the working alliance inventory. *Journal of Counseling Psychology, 36*, 223–233.

James, I. A., Blackburn, I.-M., Reichelt, F. K., Garland, A., & Armstrong, P. (2001). *Manual of the Revised Cognitive Therapy Scale (CTS-R).* Newcastle upon Tyne: UK.

Kay, S. R., Fiszbein, A., & Opler, L. A (1987). The Positive and Negative Syndrome Scale (PANSS) for schizophrenia. *Schizophrenia Bulletin 13*, 261–276.

Lazarus, R. S., & Folkman, S. (1984). *Stress, coping, and adaptation.* New York, NY: Springer.

Leclerc, C. (1998). *Conceptualisation et évaluation d'une intervention de réadaptation visant la gestion du stress auprès de groupes de personnes atteintes de schizophrénie.* Thèse de doctorat, Université de Montréal.

Lecomte, T., Corbière, M., & Briand, C. (2008). Psychosocial functioning assessment. In K. T. Mueser & D. P. Jeste (Eds.), *The clinical handbook of schizophrenia.* New York, NY: Guilford Press.

Lecomte, T., Corbière, M., Ehmann, T., Addington, J., Abdel Baki, A., & Macewan, B. (2014). Development and preliminary validation of the First Episode Social Functioning Scale for early psychosis. *Psychiatry Research, 216*, 412–417.

Lecomte, T., Corbiere, M., & Laisné, F. (2006). Investigating self-esteem in individuals with schizophrenia: Relevance of the SERS. *Psychiatry Research, 143*, 99–108.

Lecomte, T., Leclerc, C., Wykes, T., Nicole, L., & Abdel Baki, A. (2015). Understanding process in group cognitive behavior therapy for psychosis. *Psychology and Psychotherapy: Theory, Research and Practice.*

88, 163–177. doi:10.1111/papt.12039 Lecomte, T., Spidel, A., & Leclerc, C. (2005). *Expectancies and outcomes in inpatient CBT groups for psychosis: A pilot study.* Paper presented at the Mental Health and the Justice System Across the Lifespan Conference, Vancouver, British Columbia, Canada.

Lin, A., Wood, S. J., & Yung, A. R. (2013). Measuring psychosocial outcome is good. *Current Opinions in Psychiatry, 26,* 138–143.

Nugent, W. R., & Thomas, J. (1993). Validation of a clinical measure of self-esteem. *Research on Social Work Practice, 3,* 191–207.

Piper, W. E., Marrache, M., Lacroix, R., Richardson, A. M., & Jones, B. D. (1983). Cohesion as a basic bond in groups. *Human Relations, 36,* 93–108.

Ritsher, J., Otilingam, P. G., & Grajales, M. (2003). Internalized stigma of mental illness: Psychometric properties of a new measure. *Psychiatry Research, 121,* 31–49.

Rosenberg, M. (1965). *Society and the adolescent self-image.* Princeton, NJ: Princeton University Press.

Tobin, D. L., Holroyd, K. A., Reynolds, R. V., & Wigal, J. K. (1989). The hierarchical factor structure of the Coping Strategies Inventory. *Cognitive Therapy and Research, 13,* 343–361.

Ventura, J., Lukoff, D., Nuechterlein, K. H., Liberman, R. P., Green, M. F., & Shaner, A. (1993). Training and quality assurance with the Brief Psychiatric Rating Scale. *International Journal of Methods in Psychiatric Research, 3,* 221–244.

Young, J. E., & Beck, A. T. (1980). *The Cognitive Therapy Rating Scale manual.* Philadelphia, PA: Beck Institute.

Zimet, G. D., Dahlem, N. W., Zimet, S. G., & Farley, G. K. (1988). The Multidimensional Scale of Perceived Social Support. *Journal of Personality Assessment, 52,* 30–41.

CHAPTER 13

Brown, L. A., Craske, M. G., Glenn, D. E., Stein, M. B., Sullivan, G., Sherbourne, C., . . . Rose, R. D. (2013). CBT competence in novice therapists improves anxiety outcomes. *Depression and Anxiety, 30*(2), 97–115.

Crits-Christoph, P., Baranackie, K., Kurcias, J. S., Carroll, K., Luborsky, L., McLellan, T., . . . Zitrin, C. (1991). Meta-analysis of therapist effects in psychotherapy outcome studies. *Psychotherapy Research, 1,* 81–91.

Haddock, G., Devane, S., Bradshaw, T., McGovern, J., Tarrier, N., Kinderman, P., . . . Harris, N. (2001) An investigation into the psychometric properties of the Cognitive Therapy Scale for Psychosis (CTS-Psy). *Behavioural and Cognitive Psychotherapy, 29,* 221–233.

James, I. A., Blackburn, I.-M., & Reichelt, F. K. (collaborators: Garland, A., & Armstrong, P.) (2001). *Manual of the Revised Cognitive Therapy Scale (CTS-R).* Newcastle upon Tyne, UK.

Rønnestad, M. H., & Skovholt, T. M. (2003). The journey of the counselor and therapist: Research findings and perspectives on professional development. *Journal of Career Development, 30,* 5–44.

Wampold, B. E. (2001). *The great psychotherapy debate: Models, methods, and findings.* Mahwah, NJ: Erlbaum.

Young J. E., & Beck, A. T. (1980). *The Cognitive Therapy Rating Scale Manual.* Philadelphia, PA: Beck Institute.

CHAPTER 14

Anthony, W. A., & Liberman, R. P. (1986). The practice of psychiatric rehabilitation: Historical, conceptual, and research base. *Schizophrenia Bulletin, 12,* 542–559.

Barrowclough, C., Tarrier, N., Humphreys, L., Ward, J., Gregg, L., & Andrews, B. (2003). Self-esteem in schizophrenia: Relationships between self-evaluation, family attitudes, and symptomatology. *Journal of Abnormal Psychology, 112,* 92–99.

Bednar, R. L., & Peterson, S. R. (1995). *Self-esteem: Paradoxes and innovations in clinical theory and practice.* Washington, DC: American Psychological Association.

Bentall, R., Corcoran, R., Howard, R., Blackwood, R., & Kinderman, P. (2001). Persecutory delusions: A review and theoretical integration. *Clinical Psychology Review, 21,* 1143–1192.

Bond, G. R., Drake, R. E., & Becker, D. R. (2008). An update on randomised controlled trials of evidence-based supported employment. *Psychiatric Rehabilitation Journal, 31,* 280–290.

Borras, L., Boucherie, M., Mohr, S., Lecomte, T., Perroud, N., & Huguelet, P. (2009). Increasing self-esteem: Efficacy of a group intervention for individuals with severe mental disorders. *European Psychiatry, 24,* 307–316.

Bradshaw, W., & Brekke, J. (1999). Subjective experience in schizophrenia: Factors influencing self-esteem, satisfaction with life and subjective distress. *American Journal of Orthopsychiatry, 69,* 254–260.

Brekke, J., Levin, S., Wolkon, G., Sobel, E., & Slade, E. (1993). Psychosocial functioning and subjective experience in schizophrenia. *Schizophrenia Bulletin, 19,* 599–608.

Corbière, M., & Lecomte, T. (2009). Vocational services offered to people with severe mental illness. *Journal of Mental Health 18,* 38–50.

Crocker, J., & Wolfe, C. (2001). Contingencies of self-worth. *Psychological Review, 108,* 593–623.

Davis, L. W., Lysaker, P. H., Lancaster, R. S., Bryson, G. J., & Bell, M. D. (2005). The Indianapolis Vocational Intervention Program: A cognitive behavioral approach to addressing rehabilitation issues in schizophrenia. *Journal of Rehabilitation Research and Development, 42,* 35–45.

Eklund, M., Backstrom, M., & Hansson, L. (2003). Personality and self-variables: Important determinants of subjective quality of life in schizophrenia out-patients. *Acta Psychiatrica Scandinavica, 108,* 134–143.

Estroff, S. (1989). Self, identity, and subjective experiences of schizophrenia: In search of the subject. *Schizophrenia Bulletin, 15,* 189–196.

Folkman, S. (1991). Coping across the lifespan: Theoretical issues. In E. M. Cummings, A. L. Greene, & K. H. E. Karraker (Eds.), *Lifespan developmental psychology: Perspectives on stress and coping* (pp. 3–19). Hillsdale, NJ: Erlbaum.

Garety, P. A., Kuipers, E., Fowler, D., Freeman, D., & Bebbington, P. E. (2001). A cognitive model of the positive symptoms of psychosis. *Psychological Medicine, 31,* 189–195.

Knight, M. T. D., Wykes, T., & Hayward, P. (2006). Group treatment of perceived stigma and self-esteem in schizophrenia: A waiting list trial of efficacy. *Behavioural and Cognitive Psychotherapy, 34,* 305–318.

Lazarus, R. S., & Folkman, S. (1984). *Stress, appraisal and coping.* New York, NY: Springer.

Leclerc, C., & Lecomte, T. (2012). TCC pour premiers épisodes de psychose: Pourquoi la thérapie de groupe obtient les meilleurs résultats? *Journal de Thérapie Comportementale et Cognitive, 22,* 104–110.

Leclerc, C., Lesage, A., Ricard, N., Lecomte, T., & Cyr, M. (2000). Assessment of a new stress management module for persons with schizophrenia. *American Journal of Orthopsychiatry, 3,* 380–388.

Lecomte, T., Corbière, M., & Lysaker, P. H. (2014). Une intervention de groupe cognitive comportementale pour les personnes suivies par un programme de soutien en emploi (TCC-SE). *L'Encéphale, 40*(2), S81–S90. doi:10.1016/j.encep.2014.04.005

Lecomte, T., Cyr, M., Lesage, A., Wilde, J., Leclerc, C., & Ricard, N. (1999). Efficacy of a self-esteem module in the empowerment of individuals with chronic schizophrenia. *Journal of Nervous and Mental Disease, 187,* 406–413.

Lecomte, T., Lysaker, P. H., & Corbière, M. (2009). *CBT-SE.* Montréal, Quebec, Canada: LESPOIR.

Link, B. G., Struening, E. L., Neese-Todd, S., Asmussen, S., & Phelan, J. C. (2001). Stigma as a barrier to recovery: The consequences of stigma for the self-esteem of people with mental illnesses. *Psychiatric Services, 52,* 1621–1626.

Lysaker, P. H., Bond, G., Davis, L. W., Bryson, G. J., & Bell, M. D. (2005). Enhanced cognitive behavioral therapy for vocational rehabilitation in schizophrenia: Effects on hope and work. *Journal of Rehabilitation Research and Development, 42,* 673–682.

Newton, E., Landau, S., Smith, P., Monks, P., Shergill, S. S., & Wykes, T. (2005). Early psychological intervention for auditory hallucinations: An exploratory study of young people's voices groups. *Journal of Nervous and Mental Diseases, 193,* 58–61.

Newton, E., Larkin, M., Melhuish, R., & Wykes, T. (2007). More than just a place to talk: Young people's experiences of group psychological therapy as an early intervention for auditory hallucinations. *Psychology and Psychotherapy: Theory, Research and Practice, 80,* 127–149.

Pantelis, C., & Barnes, T. R. (1996). Drug strategies and treatment-resistant schizophrenia. *Australian and New Zealand Journal of Psychiatry, 30,* 20–37.

Penn, D. L., Meyer, P. S., Evans, E., Wirth, R. J., Cai, K., & Burchinal, M. (2009). A randomized controlled trial of group cognitive-behavioral therapy vs. enhanced supportive therapy for auditory hallucinations. *Schizophrenia Research, 109,* 52–59.

Reasoner, R. W. (1992). *Building Self-Esteem in the Elementary Schools: Teacher's Manual* (2nd ed.). Palo Alto, CA: Consulting Psychologists Press.

Roe, D. (2003). A prospective study on the relationship between self-esteem and functioning during the first year after being hospitalized for psychosis. *Journal of Nervous and Mental Disease 191*, 45–49.

Shahar, G., & Davidson, L. (2003). Depressive symptoms erode self-esteem in severe mental illness: A three-wave, cross-lagged study. *Journal of Consulting and Clinical Psychology 71*, 890–900.

Sörgaard, K., Heikkila, J., Hansson, L., Vinding, H., Bjarnason, O., & Bengtson-Tops, A. (2002). Self-esteem in persons with schizophrenia: A Nordic multicentre study. *Journal of Mental Health, 11*, 405–415.

Thesen, J. (2001). Being a psychiatric patient in the community— reclassified as the stigmatized "other." *Scandinavian Journal of Public Health, 29*, 248–255.

Torrey, W. C., Mueser, K. T., McHugo, G. H., & Drake, R. E. (2000). Self-esteem as an outcome measure in studies of vocational rehabilitation for adults with severe mental illness. *Psychiatric Services, 51*, 229–233.

Van Dongen, C. (1998). Self-esteem among persons with severe mental illness. *Issues in Mental Health Nursing, 19*, 29–40.

Wright, E. R., Gronfein, W. P., & Owens, T. J. (2000). Deinstitutionalization, social rejection, and the self-esteem of former mental patients. *Journal of Health and Social Behavior, 41*(1), 68–90.

Wykes, T., Hayward, P., Thomas, N., Green, N., Surguladze, S., Fannon, D., & Landau, S. (2005). What are the effects of group cognitive behaviour therapy for voices? A randomized control trial. *Schizophrenia Research, 77*, 201–210.

Wykes, T., Reeder, C., Corner, J., Williams, C., & Everitt, B. (1999). The effects of neurocognitive remediation on executive processing in patients with schizophrenia. *Schizophrenia Bulletin, 16*, 199–207.

CHAPTER 15

Alvarez-Jimenez, M., Bendall, S., Lederman, R., Wadley, G., Chinnery, G., Vargas, S., & Gleeson, J. F. (2013). On the HORYZON: Moderated online social therapy for long-term recovery in first episode psychosis. *Schizophrenia Research, 143*, 143–149.

Khoury, B., Lecomte, T., Comtois, G., & Nicole, L. (2015). Third-wave strategies for emotion regulation in early psychosis: A pilot study. *Early Intervention in Psychiatry, 9*, 76–83. doi:10.1111/eip.12095

Khoury, B., Lecomte, T., Gaudiano, B., & Paquin, K. (2013). Mindfulness interventions for psychosis: A meta-analysis. *Schizophrenia Research, 150*, 176–184.

Lecomte, T., & Lecomte, C. (2012). Are we there yet? Commentary on special issue on psychotherapy integration for individuals with psychosis. *Journal of Psychotherapy Integration, 22*, 375.

Ruddle, A., Mason, O., & Wykes, T. (2011). A review of hearing voices groups: Evidence and mechanisms of change. *Clinical Psychology Review, 31*, 757–766.

About the Authors

Tania Lecomte, PhD, is Professor in the Department of Psychology at the Université de Montréal and a registered clinical psychologist. Dr. Lecomte has helped develop and validate assessment tools, as well as several group interventions for individuals with severe mental illness. Some of these interventions are now being used across the globe. Dr. Lecomte has received several national research grants and awards over the years and has published more than 90 articles and coedited two books on psychiatric rehabilitation (in French). She is senior editor for the *Canadian Journal of Community Mental Health,* and is associate editor for the *Psychiatric Rehabilitation Journal, Psychosis* and *Revue de Santé Mentale au Québec* journals.

Claude Leclerc, RN, PhD, is a mental health nurse specialist, Professor of mental health nursing at the Université du Québec à Trois-Rivières and Invited Professor at Faculty of Biology and Medecine at the Université de Lausanne, Switzerland. His research interests are mostly centered around mental state evaluation, design and validation of rehabilitation intervention oriented toward recovery for individuals presenting a first episode of psychosis, and cognitive behavioral techniques for psychosis. His publications also cover recovery of borderline personality disorder.

Til Wykes, MPhil, D Phil, is Professor of Clinical Psychology and Rehabilitation and Vice Dean of Psychology and Systems Sciences at the Institute of Psychiatry, Psychology and Neuroscience, King's College London. She has recently been awarded Damehood for her work in mental health. She has been involved in research on rehabilitation for many years both in the development of services and in the evaluation of innovative psychological treatments. She is the director of the Centre for Recovery in Severe Psychosis (CRiSP), which has carried out a number of randomized controlled trials into the efficacy of Cognitive Remediation Therapy (CRT), group cognitive behavior therapy for voices, as well as motivational interviewing techniques in compliance and therapy to reduce the effects of stigmatization. She also founded and now is a co-director of the Service User Research Enterprise (SURE), which employs expert researchers who have a background of using mental health services. Til Wykes is the editor of the *Journal of Mental Health* and was director, NIHR Clinical Research Network: Mental Health for ten years and is now the National Specialty Lead for Mental Health in the Clinical Research Network, which is a Department of Health–funded research network responsible for providing the National Health Structure infrastructure for randomized controlled trials and other high-quality research studies in mental health.

Index

Note: Page references followed by *f, t,* or *b* denote figures, tables, or boxes, respectively. Numbers followed by n indicate notes.

CPSIA information can be obtained
at www.ICGtesting.com
Printed in the USA
BVHW020319211222
654703BV00002B/3

9 780199 391523